SURGERY - PROCEDURES, COMPLICATIONS, AND RESULTS

OVERVIEW OF MAXILLOFACIAL PROSTHETICS

Surgery - Procedures, Complications, and Results

Additional books in this series can be found on Nova's website under the Series tab.

Additional e-books in this series can be found on Nova's website under the e-book tab.

Dental Science, Materials and Technology

Additional books in this series can be found on Nova's website under the Series tab.

Additional e-books in this series can be found on Nova's website under the e-book tab.

SURGERY - PROCEDURES, COMPLICATIONS, AND RESULTS

OVERVIEW OF MAXILLOFACIAL PROSTHETICS

ARZU ATAY, M.D.

New York

For permission to use material from this book, please contact us:
Telephone 631-231-7269; Fax 631-231-8175
Web Site: http://www.novapublishers.com

LIBRARY OF CONGRESS CATALOGING-IN-PUBLICATION DATA

ISBN: 978-1-62618-823-5

Library of Congress Control Number: 2013938082

Published by Nova Science Publishers, Inc. † New York

CONTENTS

PREFACE

The maxillofacial defects may be congenital or acquired and may be caused by surgical interventions for neoplasms. Because of the localizations of these defects, aesthetic problems may occur so it becomes impossible for the patients to continue their premorbid daily lives. Losing a part of the face or having a congenital defect may play a negative effect on the social life and psychology of the patient. It also affects the function adversely. Maxillofacial prostheses can be admitted as good alternatives as plastic surgery methods, they undertake an important duty. Maxillofacial prostheses' aim is to maintain the health of the hard and soft tissues and to improve the aesthetics of patients. But completing the process is tiring both for the patient and the prosthodontist.

There are a large and rapidly growing number of literatures on the maxillofacial prosthodontics in clinical practice. In this book, I did my best to provide brief descriptions of recent developments in the maxillofacial practice. References are provided at the end of each chapter and listed alphabetically. This book is not a textbook. For clinicians, this book provides a broad perspective on prosthodontics, their possible applications and interactions between special clinics, and suggestions about future research topics, which will be helpful to their research. I hope that, regardless of your background, whether you're a aprosthodontist or a plastic surgeon, you will find the book appropriate to your needs. In this book, there are basic principles of maxillofacial prostheses and coloring, and information on patients' 'perspectives on the prosthetic treatment'. Here, I have tried to include the importance of the prosthodontist-patient relationship. This book will be a guide for the prosthodontist and their approach to the patients.

I'm most appreciative to the editors of Nova Science Publishers, Inc., for their work in bringing this book to publication. I would like to thank *Prof. Yumushan Günay* for his occupational support too. Last, but not least, biggest thanks to my family; my husband, *Levent*, and my son, *Berk*.

Assoc. Prof. Arzu Atay (DDS, PhD)
Chief, Department of Prosthodontics
GATA Haydarpasa Training Hospital
Istanbul, Turkey

Chapter I

Basic Concepts

Prostheses are artificial materials that serve as replacements for a missing organ or group of organs in an organism. Prostheses which are applied to a congenital or acquired tissue deficiency in the maxillofacial area are called "maxillofacial prostheses."

Prostheses which can be removed and replaced by the patient are called "removable prostheses," while prostheses which the patient cannot remove or replace are called "fixed prostheses" [1, 15, 23, 33, 35].

Prostheses can be supported by different types of structures in the areas in which they are applied. By this means, prostheses can be classified as:

1. Teeth-supported prostheses: prostheses that are supported only by teeth in the intra-oral area,
2. Tissue-supported prostheses: prostheses that are supported only by the tissue in the edentulous area,
3. Teeth-and-tissue-supported prostheses: prostheses that are supported by both teeth and tissue in the area in which prostheses are applied,
4. Implant-supported prostheses: prostheses supported by implants in the bone [33, 35].

Maxillofacial prostheses are generally used in cases of large tissue loss that cannot be repaired by plastic surgery methods or by using the patient's own tissues. These large volume tissue losses are called "defects." Defects are generally reconstructed by plastic reconstruction or head-neck surgical methods. Treatment of the patient through operative methods by using his/her own tissue is called "reconstruction." Some defects cannot be repaired with operative methods, while these methods are not chosen in other cases because of certain inconveniences. In these situations, the defect must be rehabilitated by prosthetic methods [1, 10, 26, 28]. While reconstruction is a treatment method where the defect is closed with the patient's own tissues and previous anatomy is regained, rehabilitation is different in that there are no worries of re-forming the facial anatomy. Instead, rehabilitation aims to regain the lost abilities with artificial materials: prostheses [2-10, 14, 20, 21].

It is essential to give place to defect classification in the maxillofacial defect prostheses. We can classify the defects according to their etiologies:

A. Congenital Defects
   1. Cleft lip and palate
   2. Craniofacial cleft

B. Developmental Defects
   These defects are formed by exposure of the growth center – which is in charge of the formation of face and mouth structures – to trauma, surgery, or radiotherapy, and the subsequent disruption or stopping of growth and development.
   Some of the developmental defects are these:

   - Prognathism or retrognathism
   - Soft tissue anomalies
   - Chewing muscle anomalies
   - Skeletal anomalies

C. Acquired Defects: Defects that are formed due to trauma (gunshot wounds, traffic accidents, etc.), surgical excision of tumoral or cystic formations, and some infectious diseases with late period necrotizing character (osteomyelitis, syphilis). These defects can be examined in three groups:

   I. Intra-oral Defects
   II. Extra-oral Defects
   III. Combined Defects

I. Intra-oral Defects

- Class I: Single-sided anterior defects
- Class II: Single-sided posterior defects (from the distal of the canine tooth)
- Class III: Hard palate median line area defects
- Class IV: Double-sided anterior or single-sided posterior defects
- Class V: Double-sided posterior defect
- Class VI: Double-sided anterior defects

1. Mandibular defects may be classified according to the type of the defect:

   a. Marginal defects
   b. Segmental defects

   or according to the anatomic area:

   a. Alveolar cleft defects
   b. Ramus and condyle defects
   c. One-sided corpus, ramus, and condyle defects

II. Extra-oral Defects

1. Auricular defects
2. Nasal defects
3. Orbital defects

III. Combined Defects

- Nasomaxillary
- Orbitonasal
- Orbito-naso-maxillary defects

Classification of Maxillofacial Prostheses

A. Intra-oral Defect Prostheses

I. Maxillary obturators:

1. Congenital defect obturators:

        a. Obturators with hinge
        b. Suerson obturators
        c. Schiltsky obturators
        d. Meatal obturators
        e. Palatal elevations prostheses
    2. Acquired defect obturators:
        a. Surgical obturators
        b. Treatment obturators
        c. Permanent obturators [24, 30]
  II. Mandibular defect prostheses:
    1. One piece metal casting binding defect prostheses
    2. Defect prostheses with guidance plane
B. Extra-oral Defect Prostheses (Epithesis): Prostheses for the deficiencies in the face area are called "epithesis."
  I. Auricular prostheses
  II. Nasal prostheses
  III. Ocular-orbital prostheses: Prostheses in the eye area around bulbus oculi and surrounding tissue deficiencies are called "orbital prostheses." Only the prostheses that imitate bulbus oculi are called "ocular prostheses."
C. Combined Defect Prostheses
  I. Nasomaxillary epithesis
  II. Orbital epithesis
  III. Orbito-naso-maxillary epithesis [23, 33, 35]

Indications for Maxillofacial Prostheses

Reconstructive operations that benefit from a patient's own tissues and plastic surgical methods always have the priority in the treatment of defects in the maxillofacial area. Plastically-reconstructive methods are the preferred treatment method because they provide better comfort for the patient and cause less damage to the social harmony. Additionally, surgical reconstruction is sometimes contraindicated. In these situations, prosthetic rehabilitation is preferred instead of surgical reconstruction [7, 10]. Conditions that form the indications of prosthetic rehabilitation of maxillofacial area defects can be summarized as below:

During excisional surgical procedures which remove neoplastic formations, it is vitally important to control whether or not the tumor leaves residue. Plastic surgical construction prevents residue control by closing the operational area, though in cases with prosthetic rehabilitation, post-operative controls can be effectively established. In cases that received radiotherapy, degeneration of tissue vascularization and the formation of some ischemic properties are factors that reduce the success of surgical operations. In these cases, prosthetic rehabilitation is preferred to surgical reconstructions. Prosthetic rehabilitation is highly preferred in cases in which the defect cannot be closed with the patient's own tissues. The need for prosthetic rehabilitation is indicated by conditions in which the patient's age, health, or solvency cannot withstand surgical reconstruction [7, 8, 33].

The main goal in the prosthetic rehabilitation of maxillofacial area defects is the effective treatment and healing of the restored area tissues. Prostheses must fix the lost aesthetic look and function. They should also fix psychological and social damages related to aesthetical and functional obstacles. The applied prostheses should adhere to the following guidelines:

1. Should be easily placed and removed,
2. Should fix the lost function,
3. The appearance should be close to normal,
4. Should be easily cleaned,
5. Should be long lasting and resistant,
6. Should not have dimensional changes
7. Should be light and easy to make [5, 6, 8-10, 21-30].

CURRENT TECHNIQUES FOR MAXILLOFACIAL PROSTHESES

Current prosthetic research focuses on the formation of facial prostheses through computer supported design and production systems (CAD&CAM) and computer supported fast prototyping techniques (Rapid Prototyping-RP). A distinctive characteristic of fast prototype techniques is that, like CAD&CAM systems, models are produced by removing material from the main source and forming a three-dimensional model in which all layers are bound by technologies like laser and numerical audits, but not by processing. Through a stratification technique, surgeons can easily manage the formation of inner details of complex structured substances and undercut areas.

The usage of different materials, different production methods of layers and their agglutination, allows for different fast prototype techniques. Stereolithic tomography (Stereolithography-SLA), Layered Object Manufacturing (Laminated Object Manufacturing-LOM), Selective Laser Sintering (Select and Laser Sintering-SLS), and Model Generation in Stacking Ergiterek (Fused deposition modeling [FDM], Material Spray Three-Dimensional Modeling [Inkjets, Photopolymer Phase Change Ink jets, 3D Printing], laser net shaping [LENS Laser-Engineered net shaping]) are important fast prototype techniques that are commercially available. In order to form the prosthetic geometry in these fast prototype techniques, five basic steps should be applied;

1. Modeling the design with three-dimensional design programs (like CAD).
2. Transforming the modeled three-dimensional design into STL (stereolithographic) format.
3. Separating the STL file into thin layers.
4. Sending the prototype bench that will produce the layered STL file again and again.
5. Cleaning the completed model and making the secondary ending processes that change up to fast prototype technique.

There are two topographic data for this procedure: a virtual image of the area where there is deformation and the organ that will be used for prosthesis design as a donor. By taking a mirror image from the digital data, it is adapted to the defected area.

Similar to conventional prosthesis, this step involves measuring the related areas with standard measurement materials. After this, a prototype is produced after the formation of the CAD model of the facial prosthesis by choosing a nose and auricular model compatible with the patient's age, gender, and face from the digital library.

In order to create anatomic details and a profile, conventional computed tomography (CT), Cone-beam Computed Tomography (KIBT), Magnetic Resonance Imaging (MRI), and computer-assisted medical imaging techniques and laser surface scanners and Optical System (OSS) are used. The created digital models are transferred to CAD&CAM and fast prototyping technologies in order to form successful prototypes for extraoral facial prostheses with good contours and tissue adaptation.

Laser digital scanner systems like Facia Laser Surface Scanner (University College London), ATOS (GOM), Polhemus Fast Scan (Polhemus), and VIVID 700 (Minolta) provide very clear topographic data without radiation exposure. In this way, the distortion and mistakes caused by the physical properties of the measurement materials are eliminated beause the data are collected without touching the tissues.

There are many data that evaluate the compatibility in the usage and combination of different laser surface scanners, CAD softwares, and many fast prototyping systems for preparation of facial prostheses.

Even though in the recent years SLA (stereolithography) technology is a popular method for facial prostheses because of its advantages, only a resin prototype of the facial prosthesis can be produced in this method, and because it cannot be directly used with silicone, it should be turned into wax form. Of course at this level, mistakes in prosthesis and elongation of delivery time are unavoidable. At this point, with SLS (selective laser sintering) technology which has recently been used in medical fields, wax prototypes of facial prostheses can be prepared and problems in SLA can be eliminated.

It is believed that it the future, facial prostheses will be prepared by directly freezing the silicone molds. Besides the preparation of facial prostheses, in the planning of the maxillofacial surgery operation, determination of the implant area, surgical stent preparation, and creation of personal facial and dental implants, models from CAD&CAM and fast prototype are used.

With these recent technologies, bone data from CT and facial data collected by laser surface scanners are united, while implant guides are prepared for creating the most compatible cranio-facial implant with the CAD&CAM technique [3, 4, 11-13, 15-18, 19, 21, 22, 26, 27, 29, 31-34]

REFERENCES

[1] Academy of Denture Prosthetics. (1989). Principles, concepts, and practices in prosthodontics. *Journal of Prosthet Dent, 61*, 88-109.

[2] Anderson, J. D. (1990). Implants in the treatment of the maxillofacial patient. *Int J of Prosthodont, 3*, 20-27.

[3] Antopoulou, II., Montgomery, P. C., Wesley, P. & Lemon, J. C. (2006). Digital imaging in the fabrication of ocular prostheses. *J Prosthet Dent, 95*, 327-30.

[4] Asar, N. V., Yazıcıoglu, H., Yaluğ, S. & Yılmaz, C. (2008). Implant supported facial prostheses. *Journal of Dentistry Faculty of Gazi University*, *25*, 41-49.

[5] Bell, W. T., Chalian, V. A. & Moore, B. K. (1985). Polydimethyl Siloxane Materials in Maxillofacial Prosthetics: Evaluation and Comparison of Physical Properties, *J Proshet Den, 54*, 404-410.

[6] Bellamy, K., Limbert, G., Waters, M. G. & Middleton, J. (2003). An elastomeric material for facial prostheses: synthesis, experimental and numerical testing aspects. *Biomaterials*, *24*, 5061-6.

[7] Beumer III, J., Curtıs, T. A. & Fırtell, D. N. (1979). *Maxillofacial Rehabilitation. Prosthodontic and Surgical Considerations*. St Louis: The C.V. Mosby Co.

[8] Chalian, V. A., Drane, J. B. & Standish, S. M. (1971). *Maxillofacial Prosthetics. Multidisciplinary Practice,* Baltimore: The Williams & Wilkins Co.

[9] Chalian, V. A. & Phillips, R. W. (1974). Materials in maxillofacial prosthetics. *J Biomed Mater Res*, *8*, 349-63.

[10] Chang, T., Garret, N., Roumanas, E. & Beumer, J. (2005). Treatment satisfaction with facial prostheses. *J Prosthet Dent*, *94*, 275-80.

[11] Cheah, C., Chua, C., Tan, K. & Teo, C. (2003). Integration of laser surface digitizing with CAD-CAM techniques of developing facial prostheses. Part 1: design and fabrication of prosthesis replicas. *Int J Prosthodont*, *16*, 435-41.

[12] Chin, K., Margolin, C. B. & Finger, P. T. (2006). Early ocular prosthesis insertion improves quality of life after enucleation. *Optometry*, *77*, 71-5.

[13] Ciocca, L. & Scotti, R. (2004). CAD-CAM generated ear cast by means of a laser scanner and rapid prototyping machine. *J Prosthed Dent*, *92*, 591-5.

[14] Craig, R. G. & Ward, M. L. (1997). *Restorative Dental Materials*. St. Louis: Mosby Publishing.

[15] Curtis, T. A. (1967). Treatment planning for intraoral maxillofacial prosthetics for cancer patients. *J of Prosthet Dent*, 18, 70-72.

[16] Goiato, M. C., Pesqueira, A. A., Ramos da Silva, C. & Gennari Filho, H. (2009). Patient satisfaction with maxillofacial prosthesis. Literature review. *J Plast Reconstr Aesthet Surg*, *62*, 175-80.

[17] Goiato, M. C., Fernandes, A. U. R., Santos, D. M. & Brão, V. A. (2007). Positioning of magnets on multiple/sectional maxillofacial prosthesis. *J Contemp Dent Pract*, *8*, 101-7.

[18] Goiato, M. C., Mancuso, D. N. & Sandefeld, M. L. M. M. (2005). Aesthetic and functional ocular rehabilitation. *Oral Oncology Extra*, *41*, 162-4.

[19] Günay, Y., Gürbüz, A. & Pamuk, S. (1991). The design of removable part of orbital ocular prosthesis. *J Istanbul Univer Faculty of Dentistry*, *25*, 201-5.

[20] Haug, S. P., Andres, C. J., Brown, D. T. & Bernal, G. (1992) Effects of environmental factors on maxillofacial elastomers: Part II . Report of Survey. *J Prosthet Dent*, *68*, 519-22.

[21] Jacops, P. F. (1992). *Rapid Prototyping & Manufacturing: Fundamental of StereoLithography*. 1st ed. Dearborn, Michigan; McGraw-Hill Inc.

[22] Karayazgan, B., Günay, Y., Atay, A. & Noyun, F. (2007). Facial defects restored with extraoral implant supported prostheses. *J Craniofac Surg*, *18*, 1086-90.

[23] Keskin, H. & Özdemir, T. (1995). *Maxillofacial Prostheses*. Istanbul: Istanbul Univercity Press.

[24] Keyf, F. (2001). Obturator Prostheses for hemimaxillectomy patients. *J Oral Rehab*, *28*, 821-829.

[25] Kurtoğlu, C. & Uzel, I. (2008). Maxillofacial Materials From to Past. *J Cumhuriyet Univ. Fac. Dentistry*, *11*, 140-4.

[26] Mathews, M. F., Smith, R. M., Sutton, A. J. & Hudson, R. (2000). The ocular impression: a review of the literature and presentation of an alternate technique. *J Prosthodont*, *9*, 210-6.

[27] Mack, P. J. (1989). Denture soft linings: materials available. *Aust Dent J*, 34, 517-21.

[28] McKinstry, R. E. (1995). *Fundamentals of Facial Prosthetic*. Arlington: ABI Professional Publications.

[29] Nagao, M., Sohmura, T., Kinuta, S., Kojima, T., Wakabayashi, K., Nakamura, T. & Takahashi, J. (2001). İntegration of 3-D shapes of dentition and facial morphology using a high-speed laser scanner. *Int J Prosthodont*, *14*, 497-503.

[30] Okubo, S. R., Kanawati, A., Richards, M. W. & Childress, S. (1998). Evaluation of Visual and Instrument Shade Matching. *J Prosthet Dent*, *80*, 642-8.

[31] Parr, G. R., Tharp, G. E. & Rahn, A. O. (1989). Prosthodontic principles in the framework design of maxillary obturators prostheses. *J of Prosthet Dent*, *62*, 205-207.

[32] Patil, S. B., Meshramkar, R., Naveen, B. H. & Patil, N. P. (2008). Ocular prosthesis: a brief review and fabrication of an ocular prosthesis for a geriatric patient. *Gerodontology*, *25*, 57-62.

[33] Rahn, A. O. & Boucher, L. J. (1970). *Maxillofacial Prosthetics Principles and Consepts*. Philedalphia: W.B. Saunders Company.

[34] Sykes, L. M. (1999). Use of custom-made conformers in the treatment of ocular defects. *J of Prosthet Dent*, *82*, 362-5.

[35] T. C. (2011). Ministry of Education, *Maxiller Defect Prostheses* (724DC0065), Ankara.

Chapter II

MAXILLOFACIAL PROSTHESIS MATERIALS

Since the oldest times of humankind, prostheses have been produced and used to repair maxillofacial defects. There were ruins of nasal, ocular, and auricular prostheses found in the archaeological excavations of certain primitive societies. It was found that in ancient Egypt, these kinds of prostheses were made at the mummification stage after death for religious purposes [26, 35].

Excavations revealed that at those ancient prostheses were made of wood, wax, ceramic, silver, and gold plates as their main materials. For example, for ocular prostheses, a convex shape was given to the metal, which was painted in suitable colors and lined with enamel. Unfortunately, for auricular and nasal prostheses, the only suitable prosthetic material was metal in those periods. The biggest disadvantage of the metal prostheses was their unnatural colors.

One of the most interesting facts regarding the retention of these prostheses is that elastic bandages were used to immobilize the helmet and face mask [19, 22, 23, 26].

Successful rehabilitation with facial prostheses is generally achieved by sticking to principles of facial harmony, color, adaptation, sealability, and biocompatibility. These characteristic properties are directly related to material preference.

Materials chosen and widely used in recent years for their advanced physical properties in order to restore facial anatomy are polymethyl methacrylate, polyvinyl chloride, polyethylene, polyurethane, and silicones.

Heat-Polymerized Acrylic Resins

Room temperature vulcanized (RTV) temperature-vulcanized (HTV) silicones are the most widely used materials in maxillofacial prostheses.

Polyvinyl Chloride and Copolymers

These materials were very popular for a long time as they are flexible, suitable for intrinsic and extrinsic paint, and have an aesthetic appeal. However, these materials are easily affected by atmospheric phenomena and lose their visual quality through exposure to ozone, UV rays, and peroxides.

1. Silicone Elastomers

The biggest disadvantage of using silicone material is that it loses its original color through exposure to ultraviolet rays, air pollution, temperature changes, and humidity. This change in the color reduces the usage period of the prostheses and spoils the patient's aesthetic. RTV silicones like Silastic 382, Silastic 386, Silastic 399, Cosmesil, Silastic MDX-4-4210 and MDX-4-4515 are currently the most widely used elastomers. There are also newly generated organo-silicon prosthesis materials on the market (MF-606, A-2000 ve A-2186).

No matter what materials are used, the prosthesis' thin edges should have high resistance against breaking and tearing, and must be able to mimic the patient's movements and soft tissues. Additionally, in order to be easily painted and manipulated, the prosthesis material's viscosity should be low.

A. Heat Vulcanized Silicones

Silicones vulcanized with heat are widely used in the making of maxillofacial prostheses. Vulcanization mechanism are formed through an additional reaction. A component of heat vulcanized silicones is polydimethylvnyl siloxane copolymer, which contains 0.5% vinyl side chains, 2,4-diclorbenzol peroxide as an initiator, and silica filler which is formed by methylsilane.

Vulcanization is a process of thermal decomposition of the initiator in order to shape free radicals with cross-bonded copolymer in a three-dimensional structure. The vulcanization procedure temperature is 220 ºC and metal muffles are used. Copolymer provides a high viscosity solid plastic. Pigments are included in the polymer with cylindrical shafts. Although pigmentation and processing are very difficult, it can provide perfect prosthetic results.

B. Room-Temperature Vulcanized Silicones

RTV (room-temperature vulcanized) silicones became popular not only because of their good physical properties but also because they are easily processed. The physical properties of RTV silicones are good, processing and colorization are easy, and they provide opportunities to use gypsum muffles. Physical and mechanic properties of these materials are still being improved. They corrode fast but not to such a degree that would impede their use for maxillofacial prostheses. RTV silicones are similar to silicone measurement materials because that they contain vinyl and hydrite siloxanes and they are polymerised by cloroplatinic acid catalysts [8, 10-12, 22, 27, 28, 31].

Experimental Elastomers

Various elastomers are researched for possible maxillofacial prosthesis materials, such as aliphatic polyurethanes, chlorinated polyethylene, silpenilen polymers, organophosphazenes, butadiene-styrene, butadiene-krilonitril, and silicone-PMMA block copolymers.

Polyurethane elastomers are materials that can gain different characteristics when the range of the other included materials change. In the presence of a catalyst, binding occurs with the isocyanate and hydroxyl groups. The amount of isocyanate defines the physical properties. Adjusting ratios through the usage of a catalyst and other components is difficult and this condition may cause false results. Moreover, this material shows properties incompatible with agglutination agents. Its advantages are that it is compatible with extrinsic and intrinsic coloring and the available for shaping the thin prosthesis edges. The cost of acrylic resin is low and it is easily found, but it is not flexible enough, disturbing a patient's aesthetic and comfort. Silicone elastomers were first used in facial prostheses by Barnhart [23]. They are still preferred for their chemical stability, resistance, aesthetic superiority, and the ease with which they are manipulated [4, 12, 22].

Physical Properties of Maxillofacial Prosthesis Materials

Heat vulcanized (HTV) silicones have the highest tension resistance (59.8 kg/ cm^2) while polyurethane has the lowest (8.52 kg/cm^2). Other materials have 30% less tension resistance than HTV silicones. When patients remove their prostheses, as there will be high tensile strength, tension resistance becomes an important physical property. There is much research effort devoted to changing the forcing-stress properties of maxillofacial materials for adaptation to live facial tissue. Medical class silicone adhesives are united with various ratios of RTV base.

The long term resistance of maxillofacial prosthesis materials is one week and prostheses can be easily torn in short time or may lose their color. These impairments may be due to various environmental factors:

a. Exposure to the ultraviolet component of the natural sunlight,
b. Wetting and drying of elastomers,
c. Surface abrasions due to application and removal of the cosmetics [4, 5, 8, 13, 14, 20, 21, 24, 25, 27, 30, 31]

2. Soft Lining Materials

Under ideal circumstances, chewing forces are transmitted to the bone by healthy teeth that are tightly held with periodontal attachments. Usage of soft lining materials is useful for the normal continuation of biologic cell activity in the support cells under the prosthesis base plaque and to avoid pain and excessive pressure. The chief motivation in the usage of soft lining material is that while the material is becoming deformed, it absorbs the energy due to the material's resilience. As a result, clinically, the energy is not absorbed by support tissues inside the mouth, but rather is absorbed by the soft lining material. Soft lining material lets the stress spread on the surface uniting the mucosa and soft lining but reduces the forces that are transmitted.

Soft lining materials should have a thickness between 2-3mm in order to adequately spread the stress. In patients who, for various reasons, become completely edentulous, chewing forces are transmitted through artificial teeth, exposing the oral mucoperiosteum to these forces. As a result of the change in these tissue functions, chewing efficiency reduces and the possibility of pathologic changes increases.

1. Excessive stress causes bone resorption and ulceration of the traumatic mucosa.
2. In conditions like these, soft lining materials are used to restore some negative factors in the bone and mucosa of full prosthesis and to reduce the pressure within the supportive tissues.
3. It has been shown that soft lining materials have properties of absorbing the shock and making the stress uniform.
4. Soft lining materials revert back to their previous shape without being deformed, while the absorbed energy is released more slowly.

Soft lining materials were first conceived and used in the second half of 19th century. At first, natural rubber was used in 1869 as a soft lining material. In the late 1950s and beginning of the 1960s, tissue therapy, surgery lining splints, and tissue modifiers for stabilization of the recording plates were introduced and used as functional impression materials. More durable soft lining materials were also starting to be used.

There has been much research regarding soft lining materials and there are existing recommendations about the ideal properties of soft lining materials for maxillofacial prostheses:

Ideal Properties Required in Soft Lining Material

1. It should be easily applied.
2. Should be permanently stuck to a hard base material.
3. It should permanently keep its softness and flexibility.
4. It shape, volume, and size should not change over time.
5. Under the force of chewing, it should not be smashed or destroyed and there should not be any breaking or cracking.
6. Its color should be stable.
7. Its taste and smell should not be bad.
8. It should not absorb water and must not have porosity that will cause microorganisms to shelter therein.
9. There should not be any harmful chemicals or materials in it.
10. It should not cause allergic reactions and irritation in the support tissues.
11. The prosthesis should be soft and flexible even with minimal thickness in order to minimize base plate resistance.
12. It should be easily cleaned and must be resistant to abrasion.

13. It should be easily processed and polished.
14. It should not be affected by bacteria, fungi, or other metabolites.
15. Prostheses should not spoil the tissue base's structure, weaken the base, or cause distortion in the base.
16. It should be capable of getting wet, have enough mechanical persistence, and have suitable viscosity.
17. Prostheses must be made from the same material as the base and be easily attached to attach the base.

Properties of Soft Lining Materials:

Cases in which soft lining materials are used:

1. In lower full prosthesis cases wherein advanced senile atrophy is evident,
2. In cases of bilateral undercut,
3. In cases where the medium palatine raphe is hard, there are 1-3 foramen on the crest top, genial tubercles, mandibular tori, and sharp mylohyoid ridges,
4. In single prosthesis cases,
5. In cases with knife back alveolar crests,
6. In patients who are hyperemic, with loose mucosa and less mucoperiosteal tissue thickness due to age,
7. In prosthetic implant therapy,
8. In implant-supported free end cases and conditions in which a bar is used,
9. In maxillofacial defect prostheses,
10. In cases of congenital or acquired defects,
11. In elastic gingiva mask preparation,
12. For patients who underwent radiotherapy,
13. As half-permanent lining materials,
14. As functional measurement materials,
15. In cases of dry mouth,
16. In order to avoid the potential negative effects of systemic diseases on support tissues,
17. In Bruxism cases,
18. In cases of recent surgical operation and on bone, mucosa, or skin grafts,

19. For surgical purposes (including restoration of facial tissues, mouth guards and tissue healing soft overlay prostheses).

Advantages of Soft Lining Materials:

1. It increases the holding power.
2. By absorbing the excess pressure, it reduces the resorption.
3. By stimulating the blood flow in the support tissues, it increases the speed of healing for bodily tissues.
4. It provides the continuation of biologic activities of the support tissues under the prosthetic base plate.
5. Soft lining materials in the mandibular prosthesis improve chewing performance, biting power, and the chewing rhythm of the patient.

Disadvantages of Soft Lining Materials:

1. Over time, they get harder and lose their flexibility. This condition is seen more in the acrylic materials.
2. The prosthetic may separate, breaking or tearing from the hard base material.
3. They may cause a break in the prosthetic base supporting the soft lining tissue. The reason for this is not the reduction in the thickness of the prosthetic base, but rather the solvent effect of the silicone adhesive and soft acrylic monomer.
4. They absorb water, causing them to change color.
5. There is often difficulty in construction and maintaining reasonable cost.
6. They become dirtied faster than the hard base material and they are more difficult to clean.
7. Fungi reproduction and surface white point may be evident.

Classification of the Soft Lining Materials:

How they are prepared:

Room Temperature (R.T.V.)

Soft lining materials prepared in the mouth are used for improving the comfort and adaptation of the prosthesis for a period of a few weeks, until the old prosthesis is re-constructed or lined permanently. They are mixed in the beginning of the process and then made to polymerize inside the patient's mouth.

Generally, there are two kinds of material used in this procedure:

a. Materials which have poly(ethyl methacrylate) and the peroxide initiator in its powder and aromatic esters, as well as ethanol and a tertiary amine in its liquid.
b. Materials which have plasticizers and peroxide initiators like poly(ethyl methacrylate) and ethyl glycolate in its powder and have methyl methacrylate and tertiary amine in its liquid.

The soft lining materials that polymerize inside the patient's mouth are easy to use but they lose their properties in a short time. After the usage of these linings, there is a loss of resilience in the material, a breaking of the connections with the old prosthetic base, poor color stability, and an accumulation of food and smell. Besides that, the additional materials used for the activation in the auto-polymerized materials may be an irritant for the bodily tissues.

Heat (H.T.V.)

These materials are formed in the laboratory, similar to the production of the prosthesis base. There are various processes that may be used to attain these materials.

Aim of Soft Lining Material Usage:

Temporary Lining Materials

Temporary soft lining materials are prepared at room temperature and their usage period is generally a few weeks. They provide the comfort and the conformity of previous prostheses until the original prosthesis is reconstructed or permanent lining is made. The viscoelastic properties and especially the ability to equally distribute chewing forces to mucosa are important.

Garcia L. T. and Jones J. D. [12] define short-term usage soft lining materials as tissue organizers and temporary soft linings that are used after surgical and diagnostic procedures for placing immediate and transitional prostheses.

Tissue organizers are very fluid when they are first applied; they require 15-20 min in order to gain plastic properties. Over time, they attain a very viscous state, when they can respond to changes in the mucosa under the prosthesis. They are fluid under a static load, but elastic under an intermittent load. It is reported that tissues under the prosthesis have a massaging effect and that they increase the blood flow.

Acrylic gels are an example of modern materials. An acrylic gel can be made by mixing swellable acrylic pieces with alcohol. For this purpose, poly(methyl methacrylate) is not suitable. Instead, poly(ethyl methacrylate) or isobutyl methacrylate copolymers are used.

There is no polymerization reaction during the hardening of the gel; only outer polymer chain spreading is seen between the subsequent particles. When powder and liquid are mixed, powder molecules swell with the absorption of the ethanol. Chains open with Van der Waals force. When homogeneity is obtained, the mass hardens with alcohol, and polymer chains take part in the shaper matrix.

Intermediate lining materials

Intermediate lining materials are used for 6 months. Intermediate linings are made from plasticized acrylic.

Permanent lining materials

Çalıkocaoğlu S. [7] mentions that soft linings are cooked under heat and their approximate lives are between 6 months and 5 years.

Long-time linings are considered by Garcia L. T. and Jones J. D. to be those which are used for 1 year or longer [12]. This type of soft lining material is named as permanent because of its long life.

Permanent linings are used in patients for whom surgery is not required, who have significant undercuts or weak residual alveolar crests anatomy, like knife edge crests. Soft lining usage increases the tolerance to the pain caused by hard based prosthesis usage in the tissues. In a patient who has prosthesis stomatitis due to *C. Albicans,* usage of soft lining materials may increase the yeast number which may cause an increase in the disease of the tissue [2, 12].

Taxonomy of Soft Lining Materials According to Chemical Structure:

Soft lining materials are divided into four groups according to their chemical structures:

1. Latex (natural rubber) and its derivatives
2. Polyvinyl resins
3. Soft acrylics
4. Silicone-based materials

Soft lining materials used until today can be summarized according to six types:

1. Latex (natural rubber) and its derivatives,
2. Polyvinyl resins,
    a. Polyvinyl chloride,
    b. Polyvinyl resitate,
3. Hydrophilic acrylic resins,
4. Polyurethane elastomers,
5. Soft acrylics,
6. Silicone-based soft lining materials.

The first four of these are not used inside the mouth anymore because of their respective disadvantages. Mack P. J. [28] divided soft lining materials into five groups according to their chemical structures:

1. Natural rubbers,
2. Vinyl copolymers,
3. Hydrophilic polymers,
4. Silicone-based compounds,
5. Acrylic-based compounds,
    a. Alcohol + plasticizer systems,
    b. Monomers + plasticizer systems.

Even though polyurethane elastomers are an ideal material for prostheses, they are not used inside the mouth as a lining material because of some inconveniences they have. These disadvantages can be listed as:

1. Attachment to acrylic base requires a special technology rather than standard laboratory methods.
2. They often do not attach to prosthesis base plate as required and as a result easily detach.
3. They sometimes turn to a dark brown color in the relatively short period of a couple of months with food and tobacco materials taken into mouth.

When the inconveniences of these four material groups are taken into consideration, it is accepted that the best soft lining materials to be used in prostheses consist of two groups: soft acrylics and silicone-based materials.

Soft Acrylics

The inner structure of the acrylic-based soft lining materials is made of a highly plasticized glass-like polymer with an inner-mouth natural glass-like passage temperature of at least 25 °C soft acrylic.

Soft acrylics differ from each other by means of the ways in which they are formed. Generally, they are initially in powder or liquid form and they are formed by the mixture of these forms. Their contents are very similar to those of acrylic based resins. The most obvious difference between them is the increased amount of plasticizers added to the soft lining materials. This change results in an increase in apparent resilience. The plasticizer used for softening the acrylic may be a free structure which is not united with the acrylic and is diffused in usage or may be united with acrylic matrix. This second method is preferred because soft lining materials prolong the prosthetic's clinic life. However, practically, these acrylics are difficult to formulate.

Plasticized acrylics basically consist of co-polymer particles that have ethyl methacrylate. As 2-ethoxyethyl methacrylate can be used, isobutyl methacrylates can also be used.

Monomers are basically used in the liquid content. Particles are polymerized with acrylates. Generally, glass-like low transition temperature acrylates are used in methacrylate homologs for this stage, but these do not have a pleasant smell.

If the lining material is hydrophilic, water can be used as plasticizer. This principle is applicable to hydroxyethyl methacrylate soft lining materials. Water absorbing linings allow the ions that crystallize to pass through the matrix over time, and hardness is evident through polymerizable plasticizers besides the osmotic pressure formation in the soft lining.

Silicone-based Soft Lining Materials

Among the soft lining materials produced until the present, silicone-based lining materials have the most desirable properties.

Silicone was first found by F.S. Kipling in the 1900s but was first used in the industry in 1930. Silicon was brought to medicine in 1947 by Alexander and its applications to dentistry were developed by Kuck in 1955 [22].

Silicon materials' resilience inside the mouth does not originate from the plasticizers, but rather originates from the inner structure of the polymer. This is why they can maintain their resilience through their service time.

The advantages of the silicone material can be listed as follows:

1. They are not sensitive to physical and chemical effects.
2. Their structure does not change between –50 °C and 200 °C.
3. They do not corrode by time.
4. Their resistance against acids and bases is high.
5. Although organic solvents cause the silicones to swell, evaporation allows them to return to their previous state.
6. They are tasteless, odorless, and colorless.
7. They burn very little, if at all.
8. They do not elicit an allergic reaction.
9. They do not absorb water and they are resistant to corrosion.
10. They are flexible and they can maintain their flexibility.

Despite having all of these properties, silicone-based soft lining materials are not the ideal lining material because there are many additional materials added to them in order to use the silicones for the purpose of creating prosthetics before they are released to the market. This is why the properties listed above decrease in either small or large increments. These materials' resilience is good, but silicones have low rupture resistance, their bonding to the prosthesis base is weak, and if they are not prepared in the proper way, they have a tendency to form an osmotic pressure effect. Additionally, they cause *C. albicans* to reproduce, causing prosthesis stomatitis. They are affected from the metabolites of *C. albicans* and other microorganisms in the mouth. In some products, there were attempts to limit the reproduction of *C. albicans* by adding fungicides.

The initial material of the silicone soft lining materials is silicone tetrachloride. SiCl4 is converted to silicone polymer with various chemical procedures. Silicone polymers are divided into two categories:

1. Industrial silicones
2. Medical silicones

Medical silicones are used in medicine and dentistry and can be summarized in two groups:

1. Room temperature vulcanized
    a. With catalyst addition
    b. Moisture vulcanized
2. Heat vulcanized

Silicones that polymerize directly in room temperature are temporary lining materials. The union and polymerization of these two component systems is the same as the elastomeric silicone measurement materials that polymerize with condensation. The biggest disadvantage of these silicones is that their adhesion is bad, which is generally seen in the binding areas between acrylic and silicone in the prosthesis' edges. The adhesive failure between the lining material and prosthesis base forms a suitable environment for bacterial reproduction and quickens the corruption of the soft lining material. This is why a binding agent is used for binding the soft lining to the hard acrylic prosthesis base.

Silicones which are vulcanized at room temperature use condensation cross binding systems based on organotin derivates, much like the measurement silicones.

Silicones polymerized inside the muffle with heat are generally paste or gel systems that include oxygen catalysts. They do not require a binding agent for binding with an acrylic base. Because silicone polymers are volatile materials, they work as adhesives. In their formulations are Siloxane methacrylate, which can be polymerized in the prosthetic base, and additional silicones. Heat vulcanized silicones form a higher number of cross-linkings and have longer clinical lives.

Silicone-based soft lining materials' main structure is poly-dimethyl siloxane. Silicone lining materials mixed with their catalysts vulcanize inside the patient's mouth within a few minutes. They also have an adhesive in order to bind to the base plate. The adhesives used in this process are silicone polymers inside an organic solvent. Silicone-based materials that vulcanize with moisture are used more often as silicone adhesives. These materials help bind the other silicone-based materials to the prosthesis base plate.

Comparison of Silicone- and Acrylic-Based Soft Lining Materials:

There are significant differences between silicone and acrylic based soft lining materials, as listed below:

1. Silicone-based soft lining materials can maintain their softness longer than acrylic-based materials. This difference comes from their main structure's softness. But for the acrylic materials, plasticizers are added into them in order to make them soft. Hardening is seen as these materials leak by time.
2. Silicone-based soft lining materials are more resistant to color change compared to acrylic-based ones.
3. Acrylic-based soft lining materials bind better to the acrylic base plate because of their structure.
4. Acrylic-based soft lining materials absorb more water than silicon materials.
5. Silicone-type materials are more elastic than the acrylic ones. Thereby, they can be used more successfully in cases with undercut.
6. Silicone-based soft lining materials allow fungal microorganisms to reproduce at a higher rate, as acrylic materials have a bacteriostatic effect.

In addition to these materials, there is also polyphosphasine fluoroelastomer, which is a half-organic elastomer made from the mastic tree. The material is produced in plates with a certain thickness and a readiness to polymerize. It has two types: soft and hard. It is possible to use these two together under the prosthetic base plate. Therefore, the soft type is used in the areas where the pain is seen the most and the hard type is used in prosthesis' edges and the base vestibule's inner face [1, 2, 4, 12, 28, 34].

3. Prosthesis Base Resins

In the middle 19th century, the first polymer-based material used as a prosthesis base material was a vulcanized rubber prosthesis material. Later, it was replaced with polymethyl methacrylate (PMMA).

In the following years, polyvinyl acrylic and polyamides were used in the production of the prosthesis bases. Urethane dimethylacrylate, which is activated by light, was recommended for prosthesis base production. But as none of these materials have the physical and aesthetic properties that PMMA have, PMMA is used widely.

Dental resins should provide the following properties:

1. They should have the transparency which allows them to imitate the mouth tissues they will replace and they should be paintable and colorable for this same purpose.
2. There should not be any change in the view inside and outside the mouth, and there should be no color change.
3. They should not expand, shrink, or tear.
4. They should provide enough resistance during normal use.
5. They should not be permeable to mouth liquids, as this may cause bad smell and taste.
6. Foods and other materials taken into mouth should not stick to the resins.
7. They should be tasteless and odorless. They should not be toxic or irritable to mouth tissues.
8. They should not dissolve in the mouth liquids or liquids taken into the mouth.
9. They should be light and they should conduct heat.
10. If it is thermoplastic resin, its softening temperature should be higher than a hot food or drink's temperature.
11. They should be easily repaired.
12. Their production should be easy and should not require expensive equipment.

Up to ISO 1567, classification of prosthetic base resins is the following:

- Type 1 Class 1: Heat polymerized polymers consisting of powder and liquid
- Type 1 Class 2: Heat polymerized polymers in the shape of plastic pat
- Type 2 Class 1: Auto-polymerized polymers consisting of powder and liquid
- Type 2 Class 2: Auto-polymerized pourable resins consisted of powder and liquid
- Type 3: Thermoplastic powder
- Type 4: Light polymerized materials
- Type 5: Microwave polymerized materials

Base resins according to their types of polymerization:

1. Heat polymerized resins
2. Chemically polymerized resins
3. Beam polymerized resins
4. Microwave polymerized resins

1. Heat Polymerized Resins

Today, the most commonly-used resin is polymethyl methacrylate. Apart from this, there are also heat polymerized prosthesis base resins like polystyrene and vinyl copolymers.

Polymethyl methacrylate is a transparent resin, though it can be colored. Its biggest advantage is that it can be easily processed. Although it is a thermoplastic resin, it is not shaped as thermoplastic in dentistry. The monomer plasticizes when the polymer becomes like dough. This dough is placed in the muffle and, as the monomer hardens over time, the resulting prosthetic base is in solid, homogenous resin form.

They are generally consisted of a powder (polymer) and liquid (monomer).

Materials added to the powder:

1. Acrylic copolymer or polymer particles
2. Reaction-started materials (benzoyl peroxide or diisobutyl azonitril)
3. Pigments and colors
4. Opacity-inducing materials
5. Plasticizer materials
6. Organic and inorganic fibers

Materials added to the liquid;

1. Basic material (pure methylmethacrylate)
2. Inhibitor materials (trace amount of hydroquinone)
3. Cross-binding agents (includes glycol dimethacrylate).

Adding hydroquinone in the amount of 0.006% or less to the liquid helps the inhibition of the polymerization during the storage of the material.

2. Chemically Polymerized Resins

Instead of activating the benzoyl peroxide by heating, polymerization can be performed in room temperature by using a chemical activator. Like in resins cured with heat before the mixing of monomer and polymer, a tertiary amine like dimethyl-p-toluidine can be added to the monomer in very small amounts. After the mixing, as a result of the reaction between dimethyl-p-toluidine and benzoyl peroxide, free radicals emerge and polymerization continues.

Another difference from the heat polymerized acrylic resins is that the chemically polymerized resin's powder includes polymer particles that have a lower molecular weight.

Besides being used as repair acrylic, chemically polymerized acrylic resins can be used as base acrylics too. However, high polymerization temperature like heat activation cannot be gained with the chemical activator.

Color stabilities are worse in chemically polymerized resins than in heat cured resins because of oxidation in tertiary amines in the following periods. This situation can be prevented by adding a stabilizer or using a more stable activator in the polymerization.

3. Beam Polymerized Resins

The form of usage and physical properties of these acrylic resins, which are hardened with a visible beam, are compatible with a heat polymerized prosthesis base.

These materials which are known as the "Triad system" include dimethacrylate matrix, acrylic copolymer, little silica fillers, and camphorquinone amine photoinitiators.

Polymerization is performed with blue light emitted from lamps that can be held, like high density quartz, halogen lamps, and prism lights. As a result of the high power of the light, it is suggested that a deep polymerization occurs and, as a prosthesis base material, it can be used in measuring impression trays, food, and repair material.

4. Microwave Polymerized Acrylic Resins

Generally, in the microwave polymerization studies, well-known resins are used, but some firms produce special "microwave" resins made just for this purpose. These resins consist of a methyl and ethyl methacrylate mixture [1, 3, 5, 8, 10, 11, 16-19, 22, 23].

REFERENCES

[1] Andres, C. J., Haug, S. P., Munoz, C. A., Bernal, G. (1992). Effects of environmental factors on maxillofacial elastomers: Part I-literature review. *J Prosthet Dent*, *68*, 327-30.

[2] Atay, A., Saracli, M. A., Akyıl, S., Tukay, A. & Oruc, S. (2007). Evaluation of adhesion of Candida Albicans to different soft-lining materials by a modified technique in vitro. *Clinical Dentistry and Research*, 31, 74-78.

[3] Beatty, M. W., Mahanna, G. K., Dick, K. & Jia, W. (1995). Color changes in dry pigmented maxillofacial elastomer resulting from ultraviolet light exposure, *J Prosthet Dent.*, *74*, 493-8.

[4] Bell, W. T., Chalian, V. A. & Moore, B. K. (1985). Polydimethyl Siloxane Materials in Maxillofacial Prosthetics: Evaluation and Comparison of Physical Properties, *J Proshet Den*, *54*, 404-410.

[5] Bellamy, K., Limbert, G., Waters, M. G. & Middleton, J. (2003). An elastomeric material for facial prostheses: synthesis, experimental and numerical testing aspects. *Biomaterials*, *24*, 5061-6.

[6] Beumer, III, Curtis T. A. & Marunick M. T. (1996). *Maxillofacial Rehabilitation Prosthodontic and Surgical Considerations*. St. Louis: Ishiyaku EuroAmerica Inc.

[7] Çalıkkocaoğlu, S. (2004). Total Prostheses. Ankara; Özyurt Press.

[8] Chalian, V. A. & Phillips, R. W. (1974). Materials in maxillofacial prosthetics. *J Biomed Mater Res*, *8*, 349-63.

[9] Chua, C. K., Chou, S. M., Lin, S. C., Eu, K. H. & Lew, K. F. (1998). Biomedical applications of rapid prototyping systems. *Automedica*, *17*, 29-40.

[10] Craig, R. G. & Ward, M. L. (1997). *Restorative Dental Materials*. St. Louis: Mosby Publishing.

[11] Dos Santos, D. M., Goiato, M. C., Sinhoreti, M. A., Fernandes, A. U., Ribeiro, P. P. & Dekon S. F. (2010). Color stability of polymers for facial prosthesis. *J Craniofac Surg*, *21*, 54-8.

[12] Garcia, L. T. & Jones, J. D. (2004). Soft liners. *Dent Clin N Am*, *48*, 709-772.

[13] Gary, J. J., Huget, E. F. & Powell, L. D. (2001). Accelerated color change in a maxillofacial elastomer with and without pigmentation, *J Prosthet Dent*, *85*, 614-20.

[14] Gary, J. J. & Smith, C. T. (1998). Pigments and their application in maxillofacial elastomers: A literature review, *J Prosthet Dent*, *80*, 204-8.

[15] Goiato, M. C., Santos, D. M., Gennari Filho, H., Zavanelli, A. C., Dekon, S. F. & Mancuso, D. N. (2008). Influence of investment, disinfection and storage on the microhardness of ocular resins. *J Prosthodont*, *18*, 32-5.

[16] Goiato, M. C., Nicolau, E. I., Mazaro, J. V. Q., Santos, D. M., Vedovatto, E., Zavanelli, A. C., Filho, H. G. & Pellizzer, E. P. (2010). Mobility, aesthetic, implants, and satisfaction of the ocular prostheses wearers. *J Craniofac Surg*, *21*, 160-4.

[17] Goiato, M. C., Moreno, A., Dos Santos, D. M., de Carvalho Dekon, S. F., Pellizzer, E. P. & Pesqueira, A. A. (2010). Effect of polymerization and accelerated aging on iris color stability of ocular prosthesis. *Cont Lens Anterior Eye*, *33*, 215-8.

[18] Gray, P. H. K. (1976). Radiography of ancient Egyptian mummies. *Med Radiogr Photogr*, *43*, 34-44.

[19] Haug, S. P., Andres, C. J., Brown, D. T. & Bernal, G. (1992) Effects of environmental factors on maxillofacial elastomers: Part II . Report of Survey. *J Prosthet Dent*, *68*, 519-22.

[20] Haung, S. P., Andres, C. J. & Moore, B. K. (1999). Color stability and colorant effect on maxillofacial elastomers: Part II: Weathering effect on physical properties. *J Prosthet Dent*, *81*, 423-30.

[21] Keskin, H. & Özdemir, T. (1995). *Maxillofacial Prostheses*. Istanbul: Istanbul Univercity Press.

[22] Kurtoğlu, C. & Uzel, I. (2008). Maxillofacial Materials From to Past. *J Cumhuriyet Univ. Fac. Dentistry*, *11*, 140-4.

[23] Lemon, J. C., Chambers, M. S., Jacobsen, M. L. & Powers, J. M. (1995). Color stability of facial prostheses. *J Prosthet Dent*, *74*, 613-8.

[24] Mancuso, D. N., Goiato, M. C. & Dekon, S. F. C. (2009). Evaluation visual of color stability after accelerated aging of pigmented and non-pigmented silicones to be used in facial prostheses. *Indian J Dent Res*, *20*, 77-80.

[25] Martin, O. & Clodious, L. (1979). The history of artificial eyes. *Ann Plastic Surg*, *3*,168-70.

[26] McKinstry, R. E. (1995). *Fundamentals of Facial Prosthetic*. Arlington: ABI Professional Publications.

[27] Okubo, S. R., Kanawati, A., Richards, M. W. & Childress, S. (1998). Evaluation of Visual and Instrument Shade Matching. *J Prosthet Dent*, *80*, 642-8.

[28] Polyzois, G. L. (1999).Color stability of facial silicone prosthetic polymers after outdoor weathering. *J Prosthet Dent*, *82*, 447-50.

[29] Raizada, R. K. (2007). Ocular prosthesis. *Cont Lens Anterior Eye*, *30*, 152-62.

[30] Verdonck, H. W. D., Poukens, J., Overveld, H. V. & Riediger, D. (2003). Computer-assisted maxillofacial prosthodontics: A new treatment protocol. *Int J Prosthodont*, *16*, 326-8.

[31] Yazici, B. (2007). Comparison between motility of biointegratable and silicone orbital implants. *Am J Ophthalmol*, *144*, 786-7.

Chapter III

Defects and Obturators

A defect is a deficiency and it can be congenital, acquired, or developmental. The classification of the knowledge about defects was outlined in Chapter I.

The term obturator comes from the Latin Word *obturare*, which means "to block." In the prosthodontic literature, devices that close/block the congenital or acquired passages are known as obturators. Additionally, when there are differences between congenital and acquired passages in prosthetic rehabilitations, the prosthetic devices applied to these should be distinguished too. This is why the devices that fix the congenital passages are called "fissure obturators" and the ones that fix the acquired passages are called "resection obturators".

1. Resection Obturators

Measurement Methods in the Production of Resection Obturators:

The measurements that need to be taken before the operation for the production of the surgical obturators do not require a special feature. A standard measurement impression tray and irreversible hydrocolloid measurement material are sufficient for conventional standard measurement methods. But there are different approaches for treatment through obturators. For the production of the treatment obturator, there is no need for re-taking a measurement in studies in which a base plate of a surgical obturator is used.

Additionally, preparation of a new base plate with a clasp holder for the treatment obturator, requires taking a maxillary measurement that shows all details of the defect and maxillary tissues that are needed and will be left. According to some data, a different measurement method is recommended for taking a measurement of a maxillary defect in which the epithelization is not completed and can be difficult, traumatic, and painful. In this regard, measurement must be made with a standard impression tray and irreversible hydrocolloid while the surgical obturators' upper structure is still in its place. After that, the silicone's upper structure, which is removed from its place inside the defect, is placed in the hydrocolloid measurement slot, and with this method, the measurement pattern is filled and a perfect measurement is made with an easy and non-traumatic method [1, 2, 4, 8, 14, 23].

Measurement procedure takes place most of the time in cases of permanent obturators. Before taking measurement for permanent obturators, several preparations and issues must be considered [1-3]:

- First of all, the standard impression tray for measurement should be tried and, if needed, modified with pink wax.
- In order to increase the retention, stability, and support of the obturator, undercut areas inside the defect can be used, but undercuts which are deeper than they should be may complicate the usage. Accordingly, the number of undercut areas that will be used should be decided beforehand and the parts of the undercuts which are excessively deep should be blocked with buffers.
- The possibility of measurement materials invading the respiratory tract causes danger. In order to prevent this, it would be helpful to cover the respiratory tract with vaselined buffers, but these buffers should be tied with ropes for the aspiration risk, and the other end of the ropes should be taken out of the mouth.

Second Measurement for Cases involving Teeth:

The recommended measurement methods for cases involving teeth changes are necessary to accommodate the presence of a metal casting skeleton or acrylic base. At the same time, measurement methods are important in cases in which the mouth opening is limited.

Cases in which a Metal Casting Skeleton is Planned

A second measurement is taken by loading irreversible hydrocolloid or silicone inside the individual measurement impression tray. The defect part on the result model is filled with plaster, plastrin, putty, or silicone putty and an edentulous alveolar crest look is produced. A metal casting skeleton is gained on the refractor model produced from this initial model. After the inner mouth trial of the metal casting skeleton, the inside of the defect is filled with silicone putty. The patient is then asked to make functional movements. The removed silicone putty's defect surfaces are loaded with liquid silicone and replaced. After this, a metal casting skeleton is located. After the hardening of the measurement material, the skeleton and measure are removed together and locate on the model which defect part should be removed with a saw. In this way, the integrity of the new changed model cut, which forms the defect part and old main model part, is maintained by replacing it with plaster.

Acrylic Base Plate Planned Cases

If the tissues in the defect are intact and not overly sensitive, silicone putty is loaded to the part of the personal measurement impression tray which faces the defect, rough measure is taken, and the impression tray is removed from the mouth. Unwanted overflowing parts are removed by cutting, and additions are made if needed. For the parts that face the remaining maxillary structures, by putting adhesive on the silicone, hydrocolloid measurement material is loaded as a thin layer on the defect part and a thicker layer is placed on the remaining maxillary part, and the impression tray is placed again inside the mouth. If there are sensitive tissues and surfaces in the defect, it is useful to take the second measurement by irreversible hydrocolloid and, in order not to irritate the patient, the mixing water temperature should be carefully monitored.

Cases with Limited Mouth Opening

These types of cases are the most difficult ones in which to make a measurement. In cases of small mouth opening, the measurement can be taken in pieces. According to this method, rough measurement of the defect is taken by placing silicone putty inside the defect with the help of the finger and by making functional movements. After the hardening, the silicone measurement is removed and a 2mm thick layer is cut from the faces of the defect walls, making space for liquid measurement material.

After this, the defect wall is filled with liquid silicone measurement material and the measurement is placed in the mouth again. While this measurement is in its place, mouth measurement is made with a standard impression tray and irreversible hydrocolloid. The hydrocolloid measurement and silicone defect measurement are removed from the mouth, separately and in this order [5-8, 11, 13, 30, 37].

The Usage of Sensitive Connection in Resection Obturators and Swing Lock

Prosthetic retention on a patient with teeth is provided with clasps or sensitive and semi-sensitive connections. The usage of sensitive and semi-sensitive connections in the resection obturator is less common than the clasps. Therefore, it is possible to have a resulting good smile while having abutment teeth, with proper planning and attentive construction techniques. In Aramany Class I cases, using a clasp on central incisor tooth at the border of a defect affects the aesthetics of the prosthesis negatively. In this case, it is recommended to connect the first three teeth on the border of the defect with block crowns and to connect the obturator to the triple block by a sensitive hold. It is believed that the holding, balance, and aesthetic of the prosthesis will be better through this method. In class II, IV, V, and VI cases, where the abutment teeth are in a relatively more posterior position, sensitive connection indication also exists, though it is not as much as in Class I.

One of the most efficient sensitive connections is the “swing lock” which is used to improve the stability and retention of resection obturators. The swing-lock connection distributes the functional forces to all support tissues and makes the teeth more balanced and less traumatic. Therefore, these kinds of prostheses make abutment teeth protected longer in the mouth. Swing-lock connected prostheses are moving prostheses which have a casted frame in two pieces. The labial section, which gives stability and retention to the prostheses, moves and is connected to the palatinal section of the frame by a hinge on its distal end. There is a lock mechanism on the anterior end of the moving labial section to make it open and close. The hinges and the locks, which connect the labial and palatinal sections of the prosthesis, are made of pourable plastic and with a pre-fabric casting method by placing it into a candle model of the prosthesis.

Swing-Lock Connection Indications

A parallelometer is used for positioning the hinges and locks for swing-lock connections. Indications of the need for swing-lock connections may be summarized as follows:

1. In the case of Kennedy I, where the alveolar crest has retentive undercuts, but the teeth do not have a convenient retentive structure for a clasp.
2. Cases when there is a possibility that common clasp designs can make a functional trauma on teeth.
3. The Resection Obturators, especially Aramany IV and V (it cannot be used only in III).
4. The loss of supportive bone tissue on teeth because of periodontal diseases.
5. A swing lock connection is used to repair aesthetic deformations after periodontal operations [5, 8, 10, 13, 24].

Types of the Resection Obturators

There are three types of resection obturators with different designs, production methods, usages, and aims.

1. The "Immediate, Surgical" Obturator is placed during the maxilla resection operation and used for the whole post-operative week.
2. The "Treatment, Interim" Obturator is used from the second post-operative week until the twelfth week.
3. The Permanent Obturator is a types of obturator which the patient starts using on the twelfth post-operative week and uses all his/her life [5, 7, 11, 23, 28].

Patients with maxillary defects are divided into three treatment stages. The first stage is called surgical closing and aims for the placement of the prosthesis in the surgical intervention. Afterwards, a treatment prosthesis stage comes which adopts the fast soft tissue changes in the defect during healing and which will be used until the healing is completed. 3-4 months after the surgical intervention, the defect stabilizes dimensionally. Therefore, they pass to the creation of the permanent prosthesis.

Surgical Obturator

During the operation, the prostheses which are used right after the removal of a tumoral mass and until the end of the first post-operative week are called "surgical obturators." A surgical obturator consists of an upper structure that fills the maxillary defect and an infrastructure in a palatinal plate shape that carries it. The infrastructure plate is always produced from acrylic. If possible, hot acrylic is used, or, if the time is limited, auto-polymerized acrylic is used. There are no teeth on the infrastructure plate.

Advantages of the Surgical Obturator Usage

Among the advantages of the usage of surgical obturators are:

1. It provides the opportunity for oral feeding to the patient. There is no need for a nasogastric tube.
2. It provides the patient the ability to talk.
3. It guides the epithelization of the inner-defect surface.
4. It prevents the unwanted contractures in the unsupported soft tissues.
5. It tamponades the free skin grafts.
6. It prevents the contamination and infection of the post-operative cavity.
7. It eliminates the psychological destruction of the patient.

Surgical Obturator Types

It is possible to prepare surgical obturators in three different types. Surgeons and the prosthesis specialists discuss the operation together on the model of the particular patient and draw the advised surgical plan on the maxillary model [2-4, 7].

Classical Type of Surgical Obturator

Infrastructure of the classical type of obturator is a palatinal plate made from acrylic. Adhesion is gained by the periodontal or transalveolar ligatures. Surgical obturators are types of obturators that cannot be placed or removed by the patient. During the resection operation, they are placed inside the mouth by the help of the ligatures. In patients with teeth, ligatures are applied by wrapping around the teeth. This application is known as "periodontal ligaturing." In patients without teeth, it is known as "transalveolar ligaturing" or "peri-zygomatic ligaturing." For both transmaxillary and peri-zygomatic ligaturing, a reverdin needle is used.

The upper structure is made of gas buffers tightly stuffed into the defect. As it is a maxillary resection, it is known that these gas buffers are used for a long time. Additionally, these gas buffers have serious objections because of difficult post-operative care and mouth hygiene. It has been reported that, as intra-defect secretions and food residues are kept by the gas buffer for a week, there is high infection risk and also a bad smell. It has been reported that the limited utility of these kinds of surgical obturators is due to the fact that the infrastructure plate closes the whole defect. Otherwise, as the upper-structure gas buffer is exposed intra-orally, contamination and smelling would increase.

Spiessl Type Surgical Obturators

Spiessl type surgical obturators do not have any infrastructure plate. As an upper structure material, silicone putty elastomeric measurement material is used. After the removal of the tumoral mass, the deep undercut parts of the defect which cannot be used for adhesion are blocked with gas buffers and the rest of the defect is filled with putty silicone. Instead, the naso-jugal flap is closed. A toothless alveolar back look is given to the silicone putty with the help of the fingers. Additionally, before completing the silicone hardening, it is also recommended to open vertical channels on the obturator. Also, it has been reported that these channels will provide a drainage channel for tissue liquids and secretions in the post-operative period and additionally will help to direct the antiseptic wash solutions to the defect wall.

Spiessl technique has advantages such as easy creation, short creation time, not requiring pre-operative planning, not being affected by the discordance between pre-operative planning and operation, allowing the defect to be cleaned, and also supporting the free skin grafts. At the same time, as it does not have an infrastructure palatinal plate and adhesion elements, it gains its adhesiveness from the undercut areas inside the defect. This causes either the lack of adhesion of the obturator (due to excessive block-out) or very hard removal from its place (due to lack of block-out).

Combined Type of Surgical Obturators

These obturators are developed to unite the positive features of the classical type and special type obturators. Its infrastructure consists of an acrylic palatinal plate. Its adhesion is gained by periodontal or transalveolar ligatures. Its upper structure consists of a special type of putty silicone elastomer and is prepared at the operation time.

During its making, pre-operative preparation is needed, much like the classical type obturator. In order to place the surgical obturator during the operation, the infrastructure plate must be prepared before the operation. For this process, the patient for whom the maxillary resection is planned is directed to the maxillofacial prosthesis clinic before the operation. The procedures that the prosthodontist follow when the patient applies to the clinic are as follows:

1. Intra-oral and extra-oral examination
2. Anamnesis
3. Radiogram and pathology report examination
4. Mouth hygiene control and optimization
5. Lower and upper jaw measurement
6. Relationship record between the jaws

The laboratory steps in the process of surgical obturator preparation may be summarized as follows:

1. Obtaining a lower and upper jaw model,
2. According to the record of the relationship between the jaws, connecting the models to the articulator,
3. Taking radiogram pathology data and examination findings into consideration, predicting the approximate surgical limits through cooperation with the surgical team that carry on the operation,
4. Removal of the teeth that are thought to remain in the resection area by scraping and giving the area an edentulous alveolar crest look,
5. Marking the limits of the infrastructure plate limits on the model,
6. Obtaining the plate for hot or auto-polymerized acrylic,
7. Finishing and polishing,
8. Opening holes in the suitable places for periodontal or transalveolar ligaturing.

The completed infrastructure plate and the silicone putty which will be used for the upper-structure are sterilized by ethylene oxide or disinfected by suitable solutions. After the completion of the tumor resection, conformity control is made by trying the infrastructure plate. This process is controlled, whether the infrastructure plate closes the defect completely or not, and whether it blocks the closing or not. After the essential arrangement, the fixation of the plate is completed. For this purpose, ligature wires are used. After the completion of the ligaturing, the defect is filled with suitable silicone, which is mixed with catalyst. Before the completion of the hardening, the silicone surface (from which the residues are removed) is shaped in a way that will imitate the anatomy of the bone surface.

The naso-jugal flap is closed and it is controlled whether the upper structure flat supports the flap sufficiently or stretches it. The flap should be supported by the obturator but must not be stretched. The silicone surface can be modified if needed, or silicone can be completely removed and renewed if needed. After the completion of the upper structure, the flap is sutured to its place.

The advantages of the combined type surgical obturator are as follows:

1. It is not a problem if the defect is wider than predicted in the pre-operative period because the defect border gap is filled with silicone.
2. Because they have adhesive elements, there is no need for using deep undercuts. This is why they are easy to remove.
3. They are good guides for the inner surface epithelization of the defect.
4. Supports the free skin flaps [4, 11, 15, 25, 28, 30].

2. TREATMENT OBTURATORS

Treatment obturators are obturators which are used from the second until the twelfth week of post-operative period. They also known as “therapeutic” or “treatment” obturators because of their therapeutic, wound healing, and directive functions. They are also known as “interim” or “transitional” obturators because they are also transitive prostheses between immediate surgery obturators and permanent obturators. The base plate of a surgery obturator is often used in the making of treatment obturators. Tissue conditioner is placed after the removal of the surgery obturator’s substucture plate and upper structure silicone and after wound care is completed. By doing this, the surgery obturator is transformed into a treatment obturator and the accordance of the prosthesis is increased. The patient will be freed from the measurement process of resected and unhealed tissues.

Besides the compilation of the healing defect's contraction of the soft tissue conditioning substances, they also have positive effects on tissue healing. Additionally, they have positive effects on a treatment obturator's hold because of their extendibility on the in defect undercut areas. These prostheses can be used until the twelfth week in conditions of changing the upper structure frequently, and being highly motivated about oral hygiene control and defect cleaning.

This type of treatment obturator, which is made by adding upper structure from soft lining material to the acrylic base plate of surgery obturator, can be worn and removed by the patient. However, they do not have clasps and obtain retention with the conformity of soft material's defect undercuts. Delayed treatment obturation can be made if this obturator does not meet the expectations. It has been reported that delayed treatment obturation can be made within 10-20 after days of the operation. The main differences of delayed treatment obturation are that it can be worked on a model and the measurement taken after the obturator is removed.

Therefore, the accord of the substructure plate to the borders of the defect is perfect, clasps are used for holding, and the upper structure can be made in different ways.

Inner-Filled Upper Structure Treatment Obturator

An inner-filled upper structure treatment obturator is a prosthesis made with a clasped infrastructure plate which is formed by the filling of the defect in the model from the post-operative measurement, tissue organizer, and feeding in the mouth.

Empty Upper Structure Treatment Obturator

These obturators can be prepared empty in order to reduce the weight of the prosthesis. In late treatment obturation, there are three different methods for preparing the upper structure empty.

Method I

On the study model, an edentulous alveolar crest look is given by filling the inside of the defect with Optosil. A clasped infrastructure plate is prepared from acrylic. The Optosil that fills the defect is removed. After that, the inside of the defect is covered by 3mm of relief wax in order to prepare a place for the soft lining material. The upper structure core is formed over the relief wax. This upper structure core and infrastructure plate is united on the model by auto-polymerized acrylic. After the standard leveling and polishing, the upper structure of the obturator, which is adapted to the mouth, is fed by tissue organizing soft lining in the mouth.

Method II

On the model, the inside of the defect is then covered with 3mm thick silicone elastomer in order to form a place for the soft lining material that will be applied afterwards. After this, a pink wax capsule is modulated within the thickness of a layer. The part of the capsule that faces the top of the defect is left open. The top of the defect is punctured from here and the gap in the capsule model is filled with white plaster. Palate and an edentulous alveolar crest look is given to the surface of the plaster. After the montage of the infrastructure and clasps, the model is muffled and acrylic is kicked. When it is removed from the muffle, the open top of the capsule is closed with auto-polymerized acrylic. After the standard leveling and polishing, the upper structure of the obturator, which is adapted to the mouth, is fed by tissue organizing soft lining in the mouth.

Method III

Method III is a method that benefits by using the surgical obturator as the infrastructure plate. The upper-structure silicone of the surgical obturators is united with the infrastructure by hand and is minimized by 5mm from all the surfaces that touches the defect wall. An auto-polymerized capsule is formed on this. After the completion of the polymerization process, the silicone inside the capsule is removed and united with the infrastructure plate. After the standard leveling and polishing, the upper structure of the obturator, which is adapted to the mouth, is fed by tissue organizing soft lining in the mouth [3, 13-15].

3. Permanent Obturators

After the completion of the epithelization and cicatrisation of the remaining tissues from maxillary resection, the permanent obturator starts. It is known that the treatment obturator can be replaced with a permanent obturator twelve weeks after the maxilla resection. Alternatively, this timing can be prolonged due to patient's general condition, limitation of the mouth openness, not enough healing at the defect, insufficient oral hygiene control, or permanent obturator usage can be otherwise delayed.

This timing can change according to a patient's general condition, age, the location and the size of the resection, and is approximately 3-4 months. It is known that in patients with big defects who received radiotherapy, the permanent obturator application can be delayed up to 6-12 months due to the dosage of the radiotherapy.

These obturators which are used after the treatment obturators, are obturators which are used 3-6 months after the resection. After the application, they do not need to be renewed. Permanent adhesion is gained from the undercut area or existing teeth, much like the treatment obturators.

The prosthetic approach in the treatment of the maxillary defect can be listed in two separate groups:

1. Prosthetic treatment of the small resection: small perforations or defects in maxilla are easier to fix. Besides this, the widest diameter of the maxilla's upper structure should not be larger than the entry diameter of the defect in the palate level, and we must know that the upper structure is parallel to the entrance of the cavity.
2. Prosthetic treatment of the large resection: cases in which maxilla are removed in the middle or upper structure level, in addition to cases in which bulbus occuli are removed with the orbital base, are prosthetically more problematic than the other cases. In these types of cases, the design of the prosthesis must be made according to the size and the deepness of the defect and the supporting areas. Obturators can be classified according to the hardness of the material – as rigid, flexible, or combined – and they are classified according to their piece number as monoblock or multiblock.

The design of the obturators is defined as upper structure or lower structure design.

Upper Structure Design in Permanent Obturators

Obturators which include an upper structure prepared from hard materials are called "rigid obturators." Obturators which include an upper structure from materials like silicone, soft acrylic, and rubber are called "flexible obturators." Obturators which are made with a rigid acrylic core covered by soft material are called "combined type obturators." In the combined obturators, usage of silicone as a soft material can form an intermediate phase by easing the union of acrylic and silicone. With this aim, "Biocryl" was recommended and used.

In order to make the production and the usage of the prosthesis easier, it is recommended to use monoblock obturators, which have only one piece, in all possible cases. But in cases in which the obturator is too large to be placed in the mouth in one piece, a multi-pieced "multiblock" obturator is required. In these types of studies, slotted, pinned, or magnetic connections can be used for the union of the lower and upper structures. It can be useful if these study models are prepared in two pieces – because the defects are very large and the defect undercuts are very deep – and if these two pieces are united with package rubber during the making of the obturator. Generally, after the resection of the maxillary tumor, large volume defects come out. The fact that the obturators which restore these defects have large volumes is inevitable. Besides the good rotation movements under the obturator's functional forces, some precautions are recommended for a good support, retention, stability, and aesthetics, but the most helpful approach is to prepare the upper structure's inside while it is empty. The permanent obturator with an empty inner upper structure is produced in two different types.

Open Spaced (Buccal Extended-Pooled) Upper Structure

The upper structure which has medial, lateral, anterior, and posterior sides have an open top. Basically, it looks like a pool or bowl. The easiest way to make this type of obturator is first to make the prosthesis full and then empty it. But in this method, the wall thickness cannot be controlled. Currently, an orally-defined plaster core method is used. This type of upper structure has a positive effect on the understandability of a patient's speech.

Plaster Core Method

Originally, this method is designed for the completely edentulous cases. The study model is opened by scraping the top of the defect. The side walls of the defect are covered with pink wax with a 3mm thickness. The inside of the defect is filled with white plaster. An edentulous alveolar crest look is given to the open surface. In this way, palatinal plate modeling is made on the maxillary model with an anatomic integrity, and the acrylic is stuffed. The apparatus which is gained by this method is used in the recording of the relationship between the both jaws, tooth making, and trials. It is again taken to the muffle for forming the final shape of the teeth sequence.

The plaster core method defined for edentulous maxilla can be also modified for partial edentulous alveoli. In this method, the defect in the model is filled with silicone putty and an edentulous alveolar back look is given to it. The obturator infrastructure is prepared and brought to the level of trial with teeth. It does not matter whether the infrastructure is metal casting or acrylic. The infrastructure and defect silicone are removed. The top of the defect is opened by scraping. The side walls of the defect are covered with 3mm thick pink wax. The inside of the defect is filled with white plaster. Before the plaster freezes, the modeling is placed and the overflow plaster is cleaned. All around the union line between infrastructure plate and model, wax is stuck and the model is muffled. As the wax covering goes away while melting the wax, a white plaster core stays in the middle of the core defect. Isolation acrylic stuffing and polishing is completed with the known methods.

Though making the open spaced obturators is easy, they are not hygienic, as the secretion accumulates inside the bowl. Good oral hygiene and prosthesis hygiene should be provided for the patients. Covering it with liquid acrylic in order to fix the unpolished parts of the space is recommended in order to reduce the bacteria retention.

Upper Structure with Cover and Space (Hollow Bulb)

The easiest method for making this prosthesis is to prepare it full and then empty the inside and close with an auto-polymerized cover. However, the wall thickness of the upper structure cannot be controlled with this method. Another approach to gain space is to form a closed spaced structure, which benefits from a place covering material and then the removal for forming the upper structure's space. With this aim, materials like ice, powdered sugar, clay, liquid plaster, polyurethane foam, and aspest are used. Also in these methods, the thickness of the wall cannot be controlled. This type of obturator can also be made by closing an open spaced obturator by sticking an acrylic cover with auto-polymerized acrylic. Technical problems other than reducing the weight in the closed space upper structure are obtaining uniform wall thickness and providing impermeability. An acrylic core method which is made for this provides a solution to all these problems, but besides that, it is also difficult and time consuming.

Acrylic Core Method

The defect on the model is filled with silicone putty, an edentulous alveolar back look is given to it, and it is brought to the trial stage with teeth. The wax in which the teeth sequence and modeling is completed is then taken to the sample muffle. After taking away the wax and the defect silicone, all the surfaces that face the defect are covered with 2mm thick pink wax. Three holes are opened on this layer for a stopper. Relief wax is covered with 2mm thick auto-polymerized acrylic. The lower and upper acrylic pieces in the muffle are polymerized separately. Heat and pressure are used for this stage. By combining the lower and upper acrylic pieces, an acrylic core with an empty inside is obtained. While putting the hot acrylic in the muffle, a controlled wall thickness and an impermeable upper structure are gained.

A Simplified Acrylic Core Method

The defect on the model is filled with silicone putty, an edentulous alveolar back look is given to it, and it is brought to the trial stage with teeth. After finishing the teeth sequence and modeling, a wax sample study model is separated and taken to another muffle and filled with acrylic. In the study model, after taking away the wax and the defect silicone, all the surfaces that face the defect are covered with 2mm thick pink wax. Relief wax is covered with 2mm thick auto-polymerized acrylic. Just before the completion of the polymerization, union with the auto-polymerized core is obtained while adapting to its place on the infrastructure study design. After the completion of the polymerization, the prosthesis is separated from the model, relief wax is removed with hot water, and acrylic is filled in the space remaining from the relief wax. It is possible that this method which is described for completely edentulous maxilla will be adapted to the infrastructure in the shape of partial edentulous maxilla metal casting frame [2, 5, 13, 15].

Infrastructure Design for Permanent Obturators

The obturator's infrastucture plate is in the shape of a total prosthesis in total edentulous cases when there are no teeth on residual alveolar crests. This infrastructure plate has to reduce the specific chewing pressure by closing the expansion of the defect to the oral cavity and distributing the functional forces over the largest possible area by covering all maxillary tissues until moving tissue borders, as in all prosthesis base plates. Additionally, infrastructure design requires a more detailed evaluation in partially-toothless cases which require monoblock casted infrastructures. In these applications, it is necessary to consider functional and parafunctional forces which effect the obturator. The forces affecting the resection obturator may occur during this function because of the prosthesis' own weight, and can affect the obturator together in a fairly complicated form [1, 2, 5, 6, 12, 25, 30, 38].

Adhesive Devices Used in Obturator Prostheses for Increasing the Adhesion

In order to increase the adhesion and the stability of the prostheses, mechanic methods are required. In order to gain the wanted adhesion, in the absence of the normal structures and the completion of them with grafts, helping adhesive devices can be used.

Elastic Materials

Two types of elastic materials are used in the obturator prosthesis application.

Usage for the Patients with Temporary Elastic Material Resection

Before the making of the permanent obturator prostheses, elastic materials are used when the residue back has to be protected, for healing the mouth mucosa which became hypertrophic, irritated, hyperemic, and displaced. The self-hardening elastic materials, which are put inside the prosthesis, are appropriate for the healing of the traumatized tissues where the prosthesis is placed. The following are the special conditions in which these types of materials are used:

1. In the treatment of hyperemic and traumatized mouth mucosa caused by not-well-tolerated, bad occlusion prostheses and bruxism.
2. Frequently in the treatment of wide pressure areas of the maxilla and papillary hyperplasia due to excessive occlusal pressure.

In the permanent obturators, elastic materials are added directly in the mouth or indirectly after the measurement of the surgical defect.

1. As the fixing material and base plate in edentulous patients – if there are undercuts – elastic materials are used in the inner-mouth record fixation. This procedure increases the stability, retention, and the comfort of the base plate.
2. When the surgical resection is completed and they are removed as a surgical plate or splint lining, surgical prostheses, which are prepared by the prosthesis specialist as lined with elastic materials, are applied to the mouth. Soft lining provides the plate a tighter concordance to the tissues and protects it from the trauma. Soft lining material also goes inside the existing undercuts and helps the adhesion of the prosthesis by jumping over it.

Usage of Permanent Elastic Materials for Patients with Resection

Permanent Elastic Materials must have these specifications:

1. Must provide good adhesion,
2. Dimensional stability,
3. Permanent elasticity,
4. Low water absorption characteristics,
5. Color stability,
6. Easily cleanable and high corrosion resistance,
7. Scentless and tasteless,
8. Should be non-irritating on oral mucosa.

Non-elastic materials have all of the above specifications. However, in recent years, stable elastic materials which are close to all of these specifications have been improved. Most of these known and applied materials are silicone based.

These kinds of materials are used in the treatment of patients with congenital or maxillary defects in pressure areas where tissue undercut repair is surgically contraindicated with the history of alveolar back resorption. These materials are used with an adhesive in order to stick to the rigid part.

Inflatable Obturator Rubber Bulbs

Inflatable obturator rubber bulbs are prescribed for patients with large defects. The obturator is connected to the prosthesis by the silicone base and there is a rubber balloon in it which contains an air valve. The balloon is inflated with air. The device provides a good implement at the back of the mouth and the nose and adapts very well as the shape changes in the mouth after the operation because that it can be inflated after it is applied to the mouth, offering the possibility to use it even with very limited mouth opening. It also has features like being light and well-holding [6, 9, 11, 13, 14, 16, 25, 28].

Prostheses That Take the Face and the Maxilla

In prostheses that include some part of the face and the maxilla, adhesion is provided by maxillofacial prostheses. This procedure is performed through the usage of a magnet or a different type of slide between the defect and maxillofacial prosthesis. The maxillofacial prosthesis in which the adhesion is easily gained also maintains the obturator prosthesis adhesion [9, 25].

Springs

For patients with total or partial maxillary resection, prosthesis retention is provided by the usage of springs. In edentulous patients with mandibulary resection, springs provide adhesion and stability for lower defect prostheses with the power it takes from maxillary prosthesis, which are not mobile.

Besides the benefits that springs provide, like adhesion and stability in patients with resection, they also have some disadvantages, including:

1. They cause alveolar resorption due to their continuous pressure.
2. Mucosa membrane may show intolerance to this pressure.
3. The cheek's inner surfaces can become irritated due to friction.
4. Side movements become limited.
5. Spiral springs are not hygienic.

There are applications that prevent the springs from collecting food materials around it and prevent the cheeks from experiencing irritation.

Magnetics

Magnetics can be used for patients with mandibular resection and are made as an adhesive between inner or outer mouth and face prostheses. Besides that, in patients with maxillofacial prosthesis treatment, it is possible to maintain adhesiveness from the magnetic implants.

Magnetic effect can pass through water, plastic, skin, and bone, and does not harm the bodily tissues. But in the inner mouth usage, as it conducts continuous pressure to the prosthesis, resorptions in the maxillary cones, articulatio temporomandibularis pain and tiredness in the maxilla can be seen [1, 2, 9].

Adhesives

Adhesives are usable in patients who need maxillofacial prostheses in order to prevent morale loss because of the lack of adhesion. Additionally, it makes it easier for the prosthodontist to take records and trials with teeth. Adhesives are not recommended to be used permanently, except in cases of resection prosthesis.

Suckers

Simple suckers which are shaped according to the characteristics of the remaining maxillary structures contribute to adhesion with the condition of frequent control. However, suckers increase the circulation disorder in the hard palate and cause pathologic formations like holes and even malignant tumors.

Strengthening the Retention of the Prosthesis

Generally, the good concordance to the tissues and edge closing provides suitable retention for the prosthesis. But in the obturator prosthesis, retention edge closing can be insufficient.

As air glides under the prosthesis base in the resection area, the continuity of the liquid film is spoiled and retention cannot be gained. For these patients, even the most effective prosthesis adhesives become insufficient.

A simple device is used for maintaining appropriate retention for these prostheses. A hole is opened in the middle of the resection area to unite the mouth cavity and nose passage. This hole must be wide enough to let the air pass from the nose cavity the mouth cavity and must be small enough to prevent food and drinks pass to the nose cavity.

In order to open this hole, a 0.6mm needle is applied right in the middle of the upper maxillary resection. In this way, normal retention of the prosthesis can be provided even in cases in which the defect is too large.

As a result, the strengthening of the prosthesis base retention is related to these conditions:

1. The prosthesis should contact the middle line of the resection.
2. The contact of the surroundings to the anatomic tissues should be provided.
3. The existing undercut in the palate shell should be utilized for adhesion by a soft prosthesis material.
4. In the defects that pass the nasal septum and middle line, the required support should be maintained from the soft material.
5. An extension can be made towards the front part of the nasal cavity. Front extension should not be high enough to block the sufficient breathing.
6. The side surface should extend for the whole side wound band and upper parts of it, for the front face of the os temporal, or until it touches processus pterygoideus, and this contact must be as wide as possible.

Front and side faces should be kept long enough to prevent vertical place changes. These two faces should be higher than the middle face.

1. The pharyngeal part of the obturator starts from the processes pterygoideus on the side, contacts the pharynx wall during the function, and continues under the trachea. The pharyngeal part must contact the soft palate's upper surface. The prosthesis extension on the soft palate in the area without defect should continue with the obturators medium surface and must be limited up to the entry-exit path. The height of the pharyngeal part is limited by the neighboring trachea.
2. The contour of the prosthesis' lower surface is affected by the teeth position and the palate structures. The medium side, front side, and

back positions of the teeth are defined according to the remaining structures. Lower surfaces of the molars in the far side must not hit the mandibula in function. After the replacement of the teeth, the palate contour should be symmetrical with the prosthesis piece that covers the remaining maxillary part.

3. The prosthesis must be as light as possible and must be made with a metal frame if possible. The bulb must be prepared empty in order to reduce the weight of the prosthesis.
4. The existing teeth and remaining tissue must be protected. Every manner should be tried for adhesion, including mechanical devices.
5. An occlusion plan must be made very well for preventing the retention stopping during the function.
6. The surgeon, prosthesis specialist, and the tooth prosthesis technician must work in collaboration, giving the patient the opportunity to be treated well.

The Forces Which Effect the Resection Obturator

Vertical Forces

Vertical forces which have effects on a resection obturator can be either from up-to-down or from down-to-up. The down-to-up vertical forces occur during chewing and swallowing. They should be distributed on support teeth via occlusal rests. It is not easy to distribute the vertical forces on existing teeth because of reduced support tissues on a resected maxilla, and it requires the use of occlusal rests as much as possible. Because the vertical forces always occur together with rotational forces on resection obturators, it is hard to evaluate these two forces apart from each other.

Rotational Forces

The weight of a resection obturator's superstructure generates vertical and rotational forces from top-down. Eating and chewing sticky foods are also effective in generating similar forces. The prior precaution to reduce these types of forces is meant to decrease the weight of superstructure as much as possible. It is also essential to enhance the medial and lateral walls of the superstructure in order to keep the rotational forces under control.

Lateral Forces

Lateral forces occur as a result of the chewing motion's lateral contacts and left-right side movements of the maxilla. It is compulsory to remove early contact points and to provide a sufficiently wide contact in order to reduce the forces. It is also necessary to increase the number of clasps and reciprocal components which provide stability to prostheses. Covering the medial surface of the defect with palatal mucosa phlegm will also help to reduce the lateral forces.

Sagittal Forces

These are the forces which occur in an anteroposterior direction. They can be kept under control with the help of guide planes placed on the support teeth's proximal surfaces.

The Components of Infrastructural Casted Metal Frame

The compounds to be used for an infrastructural casted metal frame are as follows:

Clasps

Clasp planning for the cases where the remaining maxillary area is with teeth differs from ordinary clasp planning principles of partial moving prostheses. It is essential to consider certain principles before planning the clasps of an obturator's infrastructure in order to keep the forces under control which have effects on the resection obturator, in order to bring enough retention and stability over the prosthesis and to prevent the remaining teeth and other support tissues from being damaged.

Passive Positioning

All functional arms must be passive and no horizontal force should be applied on support teeth while the prosthesis is placed.

The Elements of the Infrastructural Cast Metal Frame

Infrastructure elements that are used to metal cast framework are as follows:

Clasps

In the other remaining cases in which the maxillary area has teeth, the planning of the clasp has different principles than the usual pieced mobile prosthesis principles. In order to keep the forces on the resection obturator under control, to give a functionally sufficient retention and stability to the prosthesis, and prevent the other support tissues from being harmed, these principles should be considered while planning the clasp.

Passive Placement

When the prosthesis is in its place, all the functional arms should be passive and horizontal force should be applied to the support teeth.

Stability

The prosthesis must be able to stand, even when it is not under functional pressure, and must not swing and move.

Retention

The least number of clasps as possible must be used to prevent the prosthesis from displacing under the functional forces. There are also a few disadvantages of classical holding methods of in-mouth prostheses.

The clasps of in-mouth prosthesis binding apply destructive forces to support teeth especially in cases with unilateral defects and may result in the loss of teeth by causing progressive periodontal damage.

Reciprocation

All the adhesives must have a receiver component and the support teeth must be protected from horizontal forces which occurred during the installation and removal of the prosthesis.

Support

The forces which affect an obturator must be evenly distributed over primary support areas. It is not correct to try to get all the retention and the stability from teeth. The remaining hard palate surface, alveolar crest, and tuber are also the sources of support as reliable as the teeth. Infrastructural design of the prosthesis which shares and evenly distributes the functional forces between the tissues and the teeth positively affects both the prognosis of a prosthesis and the support teeth.

Guidance and Crowning the Support Teeth

The compatibility of the guide surfaces which prepared support teeth with the entrance way to the obturator's upper structure is very important. It might be necessary to crown the support teeth in order to create appropriate surfaces, especially in cases in which the crown height of the support teeth is shorter. Other indications of the necessity of crowning the support teeth can be summarized as the improvement of the stability and retention by increasing the effectiveness of clasps, splitting the teeth with block crowns, using sensitive connections, and protecting the teeth from radiation decays.

Stability

Dentures should be stabile even when under functional loads.

Clasp Number Type and Localization

In order to obtain enough retention and stability, using the minimum number of clasps is essential. However, these large and heavy prosthetic appliances need more clasps then an ordinary prosthesis with a moving upper part. Types and localizations of the prostheses are closely related to conditions and the localization of support teeth. It has been reported that the effect of the end position which positions the adhesives above the closest and furthest teeth from the defect will affect prosthesis retention positively. Teeth of which the periodontal condition is not high enough must not be used as clasp supports without splinting. It is conceivable that using bended clasps, designed cast clasps which allow elasticity and use strength breaking designs in order to reduce the torque power which caused by the prosthesis to support teeth, would solve this problem. In combined clasps, a bended hold must be more than 0.8mm.

All environmental bars and clasps can be used on the infrastructure of resection obturators with an appropriate design and positioning. However, in case it is necessary to increase the number of clasps, it is more common to use components like embrasure clasps and continuous clasps.

Occlusal Rests

It's been reported that it is necessary to increase the amount of occlusal rests used on resection obturators and they must be wider than the common rests in order to distribute the forces on as many teeth as possible.

Indirect Adhesives

Maxillary resection obturators are in more pressure than common partial moving prosthesis and the rotation movement specification differs under functional loads. Therefore it is mandatory to determine the axis of rotation and to create a sufficient indirect retention.

Main Connector

The metal cast framed main binder of resection obturator's infrastructure is a retentive area that considered by most authors as an area reaching through defect and not related to lost palate dome and defected area.

Planning Obturator Prosthesis on Maxilla with Teeth

The size of the defect primarily affects the success of prosthetic rehabilitation. As a result of maxillary resection, the loss of tissues on maxilla is classified similarly by different authors.

The classifications of maxillary defects and suggested obturator planning regarding Aramany defects are:

The Obturators Which Are Being Applied to Aramany Class I Defects (One Sided Anterior Defects)

Half-maxilla and teeth are protected on the healthy side of the mouth. The resection border crosses the middle line. It is the most common type of defect and also known as "classical hemimaxillectomy." Tripodal planning is made on patients who have middle line resection. Support is taken from the front incisor tooth and the last large molar tooth, and indirect retention is provided from canine or the 1 small molar tooth's distal side. After splinting the teeth numbered 1, 2, and 3, a bar clasp is applied to middle incisor tooth. It is possible to get effective retention from the sides of the cheeks of larger molar teeth.

The Obturators Which Are Being Applied to Aramany Class II Defects (One Sided Posterior Defects)

In this case, a tumor makes the maxilla one-sided. The contra-lateral side and the anterior maxilla are protected.

The Obturators Which Are being Applied to Aramany Class III Defects (Hard Palate Middle Line Area Defects)

In this class, the defect has occurred on the middle of the maxilla and alveolar crests, and the teeth series has been protected. There are rests placed on mesials of the right and left first small molar and distal fossae of second larger molars, which creates a quadrangle and well-balanced force transmission scheme. This force transmission model is also known as "quadrilateral" planning. Indirect holding is not necessary in this type of resection because of well-balanced force distribution. All holding handles are located on the buccal side of teeth and receiving handles are on the palatal side.

The Obturators Which Are being Applied to Aramany Class IV Defects (Double Sided Anterior or Single Sided Posterior Defects)

The defect in this class makes maxilla single-sided and affects the front part of maxilla. Linear planning is convenient in these cases because of the specification of remaining dental arc pieces. Increasing the number of rests will distribute the support to more teeth and make the support teeth longer lasting. Placing the clasp handles crosswise increases prosthesis retention. Splitting the teeth with block crowns not only can improve the stability and retention of the prosthesis, but also can make support teeth protected longer in the mouth.

The Obturators Which Are being Applied to Aramany Class V Defects (Double Sided Posterior Defects)

These cases are those where frontal teeth and the front part of maxillas are protected, while back teeth and the important part of the maxillary hard and soft palate are removed. Rest distribution shows a triangular scheme. In addition to rests, which are placed on teeth situated on the right and left border of remaining anterior maxilla segments, the indirect adhesives placed on central incisors shows a triangular distribution. Functional clasp handles at the buccal side and reciprocal components on palatal sides must be located on the teeth which is closest to the defect. Splinting the teeth right and left side of the defect with block crowns makes them longer lasting.

Obturators Applied to the Aramany Class VI Defects (Double Sided Anterior Defects)

These are cases wherein only the anterior part of the maxilla is removed. It is a very rare kind of defect. In these cases, the force distribution scheme and rest distribution are quadrilateral. Because of this balanced force transmission, there is no need for indirect adhesion in this type of resection. All holding arms are placed in the buccal side of the supportive teeth while facing arms are placed in the palatinal side.

- In trismus cases where the mouth opening is limited and the amount of the measurement materials to be used must be adjusted in order to be compatible with the distance.
- The patient must be relieved with appropriate suggestions and the patient's concerns should not be ignored.

First Measurement

Standard measurement impression trays modified with wax supplementation and irreversible hydrocolloid measurement materials are mostly used for the first measurement.

Second Measurement

In order to have a healthy study model, a second measurement must be taken with personal measurement impression trays, regardless whether the patient is with or without teeth. It is necessary to prepare the personal impression tray and a second measurement must be taken.

Second Measurement for Total Edentulous Cases

The middle of the defect obtained from the model in the first measurement is filled with plastrin, modeling clay, or sealing material 3-4mm away from the walls. The height of the material on a horizontal plane must be extended up to the level of the remaining maxillary. The remaining maxillary is covered by a layer of pink wax in order to make space for measurement material and stopper holes on wax relief are drilled in order to make the measurement material in the impression tray to be uniform. A personal impression tray is produced by using an auto-polymerized acrylic impression tray.

Materials like base plates are not appropriate for this purpose. The edges of an obtained impression tray are adapted by straightening. It must be 2-3 mm away from all muscle connections and frenula. The accordance of tissues in defect and during functional movements (opening, over-opening, stretching the facial muscles, smiling, and "o" pronunciation) is controlled during opening and closing while the impression tray is placed, making excursion movements, and adapted by corrosion if necessary. Displacement and dislodgement of the impression tray, and if the patient is feeling pressure while opening the mouth, indicate that the upper back edges of the impression tray are too long. After stabilizing the impression tray and moving the patient's facial muscles, physiologic borders of mukobbuccal sulcus are determined on the impression tray. Early contacts on buccal and posterior walls are determined with pressure indicator paste. The patient is asked to open his/her mouth as much as possible while the impression tray is placed. So the defect's posterior lateral wall's physiological border is defined.

The defect surfaces of the personal impression tray removed from the mouth is corroded 1-2mm in order to give space to the measurement material. Melted no. 4 measurement wax is spread over corroded surfaces with a brush, and the impression tray is applied into the mouth. The defect's cut size is formed by making the patient practice the functional movements. In order to measure the remaining maxillary tissues, the impression tray is removed. And the measurement is integrated by measuring these areas with a material (ZNO ojenal) capable of measuring total edentulous crest. Besides this quite laborious and time-consuming method, more practical and simple methods can be described [7, 11, 14, 18, 30, 20-22, 24, 35, 37].

4. Ocular Defects

Eyes are the windows of our bodies. They play an important role in body image. In the medical world, eye traumas are accepted as critical cases. Cosmetic appearance is generally seen as a sign of our eyes' ability to perform their duties as the main organ of our eyesight.

Ocular defects are separated into three classes:

1. While it may not occur congenitally, bulbus oculi may also occur after birth due to traumatic or pathological causes. "Ocular prostheses" are used in this type of defect.
2. Generally, the lack of bulbus oculi does not lead to deformities in eye muscles and adjacent tissues. But in resections due to traumatic and pathologic reasons, defects affect the orbita cavity as a whole (muscles, lachrymal part, fascia, conjunctiva, and eye lids). In these kinds of cases, an epithesier with anatomical form is used as artificial tissue and it is named an "Orbital Prosthesis."
3. The epithesier which is used in restorations of cases where orbital defects exceed eye borders and affect a larger part of face is named an "Oculo-facial Prosthesis" [9, 11, 12, 26].

Defect occurrences are caused by malignant neoplasms, trauma, congenital or developmental abnormalities, and infections.

No surgical operations allow for the replacement of the eye in its place after resection. In this kind of case, eye prosthesis is required. Because defects can lead to serious psychological problems in patients, prosthesis implementation should be started as soon as possible so that patients can maintain their daily life activities [19].

In cases where eye resection is called for, the surgeon tries to minimize the tissue loss. The placement of a conformer in the hole after surgical operation is important. The conformer is used as space a maintainer. They form the eye socket during healing and provide sufficient space under eye lids for prosthesis placement [29, 32]. Also, by keeping implants in a central point, they prevent them from leaving the socket and make the new prostheses to be tolerated more efficiently by patient. But they are not used when a severe hemorrhage occurred in surgery.

For adult people, orbital volume is calculated as 30ml and glob volume is calculated as 6-7ml. By removing the eye, the volume of the orbita decreases at least by 1/5. Unless an appropriate implant is placed during enucleation or evisceration surgeries, a serious volume deficiency and enophthalmos may occur in the orbita. This clinical case is named as anophthalmic socket syndrome. No matter how large the prosthesis is, they cannot rectify the volume loss in the orbita. Because there is no reinforcement for lavatory and the upper lid, ptosis and upper lid deep sulcus formation occur. Because the movements of extra-ocular muscles will not reflect on the prosthesis, the prosthesis stays immobile [29, 31, 32, 33, 36].

5. Ocular Prosthesis

After the surgical healing process is completed and dimensional stabilities are established, the prosthesis production process starts. The region should be evaluated carefully and there must be no infection. The mobility of the tissue socket and the width of the socket are considered. It has two types:

- Custom Ocular Prostheses
- Readymade Ocular Prostheses
- Personal Ocular Prostheses
- Impression Technique
- While the patient is sitting or standing up, his head is held straight. This provides the same relations in the enucleated back surface of the socket and rectus muscles.
- The patient is told to look straight forward in order to minimize his movement.
- By appropriately mixing hydro-colloid measurement materials, it is placed into a large syringe.
- The whole socket is filled carefully without any air bubbles by keeping the eye of patient open.
- The spoon, which is filled with additional measurement materials, is combined with opposite measurement material by pressing onto the eye region. By taking care to avoid laceration, the measurement gauge is displaced by moving the eyelids.

Model Preparation and Sphere Formation

- The mold is coated with paraffin and filled with plaster.
- The mold is displaced carefully and one must be sure that all of the dimensions of ocular defect can be followed in the plaster model.
- The residual measurement material in defect model is cleaned.
- The plaster model is isolated via oil.

- The soft paraffin is poured into the isolated plaster mold and left to cool.
- The plaster mold is cut into three equal parts. It is broken from those cuts so the surface of embedded paraffin form can be seen from three different sides.
- The paraffin is adjusted and then tested on the patient.
- The sphere form is isolated with methyl cellulose ophthalmic solution.
- When the sphere is placed, the patient is told to close his eyes and then the dimensions of the spheres are compared. Modifications may be conducted if necessary.
- The paraffin form is muffled and then treated with scleral white acrylic resin.

Iris Localization

- The polished eye ball is placed into the patient's socket to be evaluated. The necessary matching must be done in order to achieve normal corneal contouring.
- The patient is told to stand straight and to look forward.
- In order to determine the position of the pupil center of the prosthesis, the distance between the pupil of the natural eye and middle line, the vertical position of the pupil center is determined and then signed with a cantus relationship.
- The iris is designed with the given dimensions. The relationship of the outer part of the iris and eyelid is evaluated.
- The acrylic eye ball is cut with equal deepness as the iris level.

The Coloring of the Iris

- The dimensions of the pupil are determined by performing shading of the natural eye and by evaluating the dimensions of light under the eye. Generally, the dimension between them is accepted.
- The first step of coloring the iris is determining the main color. The main color is the darkest color which is observed by the eye.
- The deepness sensation is created via stripes which are created from center to the outside.

- The collaret is painted with a color which is lighter than the main color.
- The last point to paint is the limbus. The color to be used in painting the limbus is generally a reflection of the iris.
- Two types of colors are used in coloring the iris. The first one is the coloring of the watercolor paper discs by acrylic paints; the second one is the coloring of the acetate discs by oil paints. Although the acrylic paints are the most preferred paints for this process, watercolors are also used. But the long drying period of watercolors and the necessary wait for drying at each phase leads to much time wasted and they are also not as stable as acrylic colors.

The Finishing of the Sphere

- The painted iris is placed in the eye ball.
- By removing a thin layer of resin, the outer corneal surface is characterized, and the thinned scleral surface is painted with blue, yellow, pink, and brown colors. The vascularization of sclera provides a more realistic appearance of the prosthesis. The fibers are adhered to the space of thinned sclera. According to the degree of the user's ability, this method can be highly successful. The movement during the adhesion process leads to the creation of normal or likable vein structure. Also, the dusts and other foreign materials in dental laboratories adhere to the wet adhesion agent and they may lead undesired results if they were not realized. The application procedure is as follows:

    1. The fibers are implemented by a wet hair brush.
    2. The fiber location is dried by vapor in order to provide protection. Drying by air is a mistake.
    3. After compilation is finished, a thin layer of acrylic resin spray is applied.
    4. When the clean acrylic resin is dried, other procedures continue as normal.

- The characterized sphere is placed in muffle and the production is completed by using clean acrylic resin.

- The ocular sphere is removed from muffle, and the refined and ocular sphere is polished via pumice and plaster.
- The prosthesis is placed into the defect and evaluated.
- The patient must learn to place and displace the prosthesis.

Complications

- Pseudo-ptosis: it is seen at a superior eyelid when the prosthesis is not reinforced efficiently by the eye. Successful results may be achieved by changing the contours of the prosthesis.
- Real ptosis: this is caused from a deficient muscle structure of deficient tissue tone. The superior eyelid falls over the prosthesis. For treatment, the muscle is shortened surgically or the resistance of tissue is increased. In most cases, the problem is solved by simply correcting the contours of the prosthesis.
- When the bottom eyelid falls, then the bottom part of the frontal surface of the prosthesis is corroded. So the force making the bottom eyelid fall is removed. The second solution is to change the contours of the prosthesis and to spread the pressure to medial and lateral regions. The bottom regions of the medial and lateral areas are shortened and the middle region is thickened and shortened.
- Entropy or ectropy lead to the unaesthetic appearance of positions of eyelids and lashes. Via some corrections on the paraffin model, the aesthetic problem may be solved without any surgical operation.
- When the patient does not use his prosthesis for a long time or after a trauma or due to an infection, a contraction may be observed in the socket. As a result of this, a loss of the socket which is necessary for retention of the prosthesis occurs. In order to compensate for that loss, the expansion on the socket can be provided by using extended prostheses. The custom ocular prosthesis has more advantages against the ready-to-use prosthesis because more realistic results can be achieved. So the forms which are similar to defect dimensions, and a realistic coloring can be provided in the eye. The careful preparation of the outer surface of the sphere allows the eyes to close more efficiently.

For adult people, orbital volume is calculated as 30ml and glob volume is calculated as 6-7ml. By removing the eye, the volume of the orbita decreases at least by 1/5. Unless an appropriate implant is placed during enucleation or evisceration surgeries, a serious volume deficiency and enophthalmos may occur in the orbita. This clinical case is named as anophthalmic socket syndrome. No matter how big the prosthesis is, they cannot satisfy the volume loss in the orbita. Because there is no reinforcement for lavatory and upper lid, ptosis and upper lid deep sulcus formation occur. Because the movements of extra-ocular muscles won't reflect on the prosthesis, the prosthesis stays immobile. Because all the weight of large prostheses is loaded on the bottom lid, this may lead a lid ptosis. In order to compensate for the volume loss and also in order to decrease the weight of prosthesis and to lighten the weight on bottom lid, an idea to develop an implant to place in the orbita has been developed. For the first time, a glass sphere was used by Mules [27] in 1885 after an evisceration. As an implant material, many different materials such as cartilage, bone, wool, aluminum, fat, vaseline, fascia lata, gold, silver, plastic, rubber, asbestos, paraffin, and cellulose were experimented after glass.

REFERENCES

[1] Aramany, M. A. (1978a). Basic principles of obturator design for partially edentulous patients. Part I: Classification. *J of Prosthet Dent, 40*, 554-557.

[2] Aramany, M. A. (1978b). Basic principles of obturator design for partially edentulous patients. Part II: Design principles. *J of Prosthet Dent, 40*, 656-662.

[3] Beder, O. E. (1968). Emergency temporary obturators. *J of Prosthet Dent, 20*, 172-175.

[4] Beumer, III., Curtıs, T. A. & Fırtell, D. N. (1979). *Maxillofacial Rehabilitation. Prosthodonticand surgical considerations.* St Louis; The C.V. Mosby Co..

[5] Beydemir, B. & Dalkız, M. (2003). *Laboratory Applications in Dentistry*, Ankara; GATA Press.

[6] Bırnbach, S. & Barnhard, B. (1989). Direct conversion of a solid obturator to a hollow obturator prosthesis. *J of Prosthet Dent, 62*, 58-60.

[7] Brown, K. E. (1970). Clinical considerations improving obturators treatment. *J of Prosthet Dent, 24*, 461- 466.

[8] Calıkkocaoğlu, S. (2004). *Total Prostheses.* Ankara; Özyurt Press.

[9] Cain, R. J. (1982). Custom ocular prosthetics, *J of Prosthet Dent, 48*, 690-694.

[10] Chandra, T. S., Sholapurkar, A., Joseph, R. M., Aparna, I. N. & Pai, K. M. (2008). Prosthetic rehabilitation of a complete bilateral maxillectomy patient using a simple magnetically connected hollow obturator: a case report. *J Contemp Dent Pract*, *9*, 70-6.

[11] Covillard, P. & Schaff, G. N. (1976). Fabrication of the ocular portion of an orbital prosthesis. *J of Prosthet Dent*, *35*, 478-481.

[12] Cötert, S. H. (2003). *Maxillofacial Prostheses*. Bornova-Izmir; Ege University Press.

[13] Da Silva, L., Ferros, I. & Rilo, B. (2004). New technologies, designs and materials for removable maxillary obturator prostheses. *Bull Group Int Rech Sci Stomatol Odontol*, *46*, 27-35.

[14] Desjardıns, R. P. (1978). Obturator prosthesis design for acquired maxillary defects. *J of Prosthet Dent*, *39*, 424-435.

[15] Gay, W. D. & King, G. E. (1980). Applying basic prosthodontic principles in the dentulous maxillectomy patient. *J of Prosthet Dent*, *4*, 433-435.

[16] Gregory, R., Greggory, E. T. & Rahn, A. O. (2005). Prosthodontic principles in the framework design of maxillary obturators prostheses. *J of Prosthetic Dent*, *93*, 405-11.

[17] Gunay, Y., Erkan, M., Gurbuzer, B. & Karayazgan, B. (2007). Facilitation of facial prosthesis placement with tattoo markers: a clinical report. *J Prosthet Dent*, *97*, 256-60.

[18] Hornblass, A., Biesman, B. S. & Eviatar, J. A. (1995). Current techniques of enucleation: a survey of 5439 intraorbital implants and a review of the literature. Ophthalmol. *Plast Reconstr Surg*, *11*, 77-86.

[19] Jebreil, K. (1980). Acceptabilily of orbital prostheses. *J of Prosthet Dent*, *43*, 82-85.

[20] Karayazgan, B., Gunay, Y., Gurbuzer, B., Erkan, M. & Atay, A. (2009). A preoperative appliance for a newborn with cleft palate. *Cleft Palate Craniofac J*, *46*, 537.

[21] Karayazgan- Saracoglu, B., Zülfikar, H., Atay, A. & Günay, Y. (2010). Treatment outcome of extraoral implants in the craniofacial region. *J Craniofac Surg*, *21*, 751-8.

[22] Keskin, H. & Özdemir, T. (1995). *Maxillofacial Prostheses*, Istanbul; Istanbul University Press.

[23] Keyf, F. (2001). Obturator prostheses for hemimaxillectomy patients. *J of Oral Rehab*, *28*, 821-829.

[24] Kurtulmus, H., Saygı, T. & Cotert, H. S. (2007). Heightened telescopic copings in cleft palate rehabilitation: a case report. *Cleft Palate Craniofac J*, *44*, 448-52.

[25] Kurtulmus, H., Kumbuloglu, O. & Saygı, T. (2008). Management of lateral mandibular discontinuity by maxillary guidance. *Br J Oral Maxillofac Surg*, *46*, 123-5.

[26] Muğan, N. (1979). *Maxillofacial Prostheses*. Istanbul: Gençlik Press.

[27] Mules, P. H. (1885). Evisceration of the globe with artificial vitreus. *Trans. Ophthalmol. Soc. U.K.*, *5*, 200-10.

[28] Nıımı, A., Ueda, M. & Kaneda, T. (1993). Maxillary obturators supported by osseointegrated implants placed in irradiated bone: Report of cases. *J of Oral and Maxillofac Surg*, *51*, 804-809.

[29] Nunery, W. R., Hetzler, K. J. & Enucleation. (1990). In; Homblass A, ed. *Oculoplastic in Orbital and Lacrimal System*. Baltimore: Williams and Wilkins; *1200*.

[30] Omondi, B. I., Guthua, S. W., Awange, D. O. & Odhiambo, W. A. (2004). Maxillary obturator prosthesis rehabilitation following maxillectomy for ameloblastoma: case series of five patients. *Int J Prosthodont*, *17*, 464-8.

[31] Ow, R. K. K. & Amrith, S. (1997). Ocular prosthetics:Use of a tissue conditioner material to modify a stock ocular prosthesis. *J of Prosthet Dent*, *78*, 218-222.

[32] Parr, G. R., Goldman, B. M. & Rahn, A. O. (1983). Surgical considerations in the prosthetic treatment of ocular and orbital defects. *J of Prosthet Dent*, *49*, 379-385.

[33] Perry, A. C. (1990). Integrated orbital implants. In: Bosniak SL, Smith BC, eds. *Advances in Ophthalmic Plastic and Reconstructive Surgery*. New York: Permagon Press.

[34] Roumanas, E. D., Nishimura, R. D., Davis, B. K. & Beumer III, J. (1997). Clinical evaluation of implants retaining edentulous maxillary obturator prostheses. *J of Prosthet Dent*, *77*, 184-187.

[35] Stewart, K. L., Rudd, K. D. & Kuebker, W. A. (1983). *Clinical removable partial prosthodontics*. St. Louis, Mosby.

[36] Singh, G. P., Sherrigar, P., Hegde, V. & Khanna, G. (2013). Prosthetic conformer as a pressure device in the prophylactic management of postsurgical auricular keloid formation: a clinical report. *J Prosthodont*, *22*, 81-4.

[37] Wang, R. R. (1997). Sectional prosthesis for total maxillectomy patients: A clinical report. *J of Prosthet Dent*, *78*, 241-244.

Chapter IV

IMPLANT APPLICATIONS FOR MAXILLOFACIAL PROSTHESES

Generally, many large tissue defects occur with surgery treatments of tumors in the maxillofacial region. Maxillofacial prosthesis application can be used as an alternative treatment for cases where plastic surgery reconstructions cannot be applied. While the retention of maxillofacial prostheses used to be provided generally via adhesive bands, adhesives in liquid or spray form, and tissue undercuts, the current treatment of an intra-oral edentulous condition is frequently conducted via osseo-integrated implants.

The most significant problem facing the reinforcement of the facial implants is inadequate bone thickness. While the most suitable reinforcement points for implant are the temporal region and supra-orbital edge, the bone thickness varies between 2.5 and 6mm for those regions. Accordingly, special extra-oral implants were designed with 3-4mm length, unlike oral implants. These implants have wing extensions in order to prevent excessive entrance of the implant into the bone [1, 2, 5, 11, 15, 37]. Also, there are some holes which increase the surface area in order to provide mechanical stability and retention. Those implants have been used in clinics successfully for a long time.

For maxillofacial defects, defect size and location, existing bone volume and quality, soft tissue, and mobility differ widely between individuals. So the number and locations of implants to be applied thereby differ. For example, while only two implants are enough for retention in auricular prosthesis, as many implants as possible should be applied for medium-large facial defects in order to distribute the pressure.

In general, the temporal bone, supra-orbital edge, lateral orbital edge, zygomatic bone, piriform bump, and pterygoid process are determined as anatomical regions which have enough bone to sufficiently reinforce implants. Facial defect treatments should be considered individually and implants must be planted where there is enough bone volume. It is important to place implants in a parallel position in order to make measuring easier. The extension of the prosthetic surface increases as much as possible the retention and reinforcement of the prosthesis. Ideally, the edges of a prosthesis should extend to tissues with less movement.

The regions where extra-oral implants may be placed can be classified in terms of volume as follows:

1. Regions with 6mm or more bone thickness: 6mm dental implants and longer zygomatic implants can be used in these regions. These bone regions of the facial skull include the anterior maxilla, zygoma, and/or zygomatic arc. The lateral peri-orbital bone generally has a volume of 6-7mm thickness.
2. Regions with 4-5mm bone thickness: a 4mm extra-oral implant or 5mm dental implants can be used in these regions. Those bone regions include the superior orbital edge, lateral orbital edge, inferolateral orbital edge, mastoid bump of temporal bone, and zygoma.
3. Bones with 3mm or less thickness: the temporal bone, piriform bump, inferior orbital edge, nasal bone, and zygomatic bump are included in this group. Usage of 3mm extra-oral implants in those regions is indicated [1, 2, 5, 15, 17, 19, 27, 28, 37, 43, 53, 55].

The evaluation of existing bone structures in the implantation region is one of the most important issues of pre-operative planning. Advanced monitoring techniques such as Computerized Tomography (CT) and Magnetic Resonance Tomography (MRT) provide monitoring of the anatomic status of soft and hard tissue defects, as well as the structure and thickness of existing bone. In cases where auricular defects would be treated via implant reinforced prostheses, mastoid bump, and air cells system, the location of sigmoid sinus and middle cranial fossa levels must be determined in order to prevent any defect during implant surgery. It is also important to have information about the location of the facial nerve canal. If orbital, nasal, or mid-facial prostheses are being planned, BT is required in order to determine the ideal implantation location in accordance with existing bone quality and volume, and to make prosthesis such that they hide the implants' locations and openings.

For difficult cases where maxillofacial and intra-oral defects are combined, stereolithographic models may be useful in order to evaluate treatment alternatives. Additionally, bone volume and bone density measurements may be performed by new CT programs in order to place implant. Though those programs were designed for evaluating bone height and the width of maxilla and mandible in intra-oral implant treatments, they can also be used for the head and facial skull too.

Implant Applications

All other treatment options must be discussed before surgery. If the rehabilitation via a prosthesis reinforced by implant is considered after surgery, soft and hard tissues in the surgery region must be prepared for implant placement. The bone regions which are important for the placement of osseo-integrated implants should be protected as much as possible or they must be resized via various reconstructive procedures in accordance with implant placement. The thickness and mobility of soft tissues at the edge of defects are very important, especially for achieving aesthetic results. Because of the muscle movements in the face, the appearance of maxillofacial prosthesis around defects, where tissues move, causes various problems. As a result of these issues, the ideal indications of implant reinforced prosthesis are prosthetic treatments of auricular, nasal, and orbital resections. In order to prevent inflammatory reactions, thin and smooth tissue must be created around implants [1, 2, 7, 33, 40].

For an aesthetic appearance of a maxillofacial prosthesis, implants must be placed inside of the borders of the prosthesis. Many guides can be prepared for this purpose. The cheapest and easiest method among them is to prepare the prosthesis to be placed in the form of a wax package so that the implants can be placed with appropriate angle and position. As an addition to that simple method, much more standardized results can be achieved via applications such as tomography and 3D modeling. Through those methods, the locations of implants can be determined by computers, decreasing false rates. Enough bone volume is frequently not achieved after resection. Especially for medium-large facial defects and some birthmarks, computerized tomography scans and 3D models created by combining those scans may be useful by evaluating the potential bone regions and nearby structures. For example, the position of sigmoid sinus and the facial nerve canal, the middle cranial fossa level, the volume of mastoid and mastoid air cell system for some patients with congenital auricular defect must be determined very accurately.

For nasal defects, especially the positions of teeth, the base of nose must be evaluated by using radiography. Computerized tomography and 3D models gained from the data of tomography can aid in the determination of the bone volume and density in this and other potential implant regions. Additionally, those applications can also be used during production processes of facial implants [2, 15, 48].

Also, skin and soft tissues should be evaluated carefully. When soft tissues covering bone implants are attached to the lower periosteum and thinner than 5mm, it is easier to protect the health of those tissues. If the skin and soft tissues in the implant area include hair follicles, scar tissue, or residual tissues from previous reconstructive operations, those tissues must be cleared and covered with a graft.

Generally, two phase surgery applications are preferred for existing craniofacial implant systems. One phase surgery procedures are generally used for uncomplicated cases such as auricular defects and hearing aids, but they generally require experience and carefulness. Surgery can be performed under local or general anesthesia, according to the surgeon's preference. Generally, the full thick flap is raised and potential implant regions are determined by using surgery stents produced in accordance with pre-surgery prognosis models. Implant regions are prepared and implants are placed non-traumatically. Then titanium healing caps are placed over the implants. After this process, the flap is placed over the implants. Following the healing, upper structures are placed over the implants by opening the upper surface of the implants. In this way, the two phased surgery is applied. If the one phase surgery is preferred, upper structures are placed directly over the implants and then the flap is closed. In the second surgery phase, the tissue flap around the implant must be thinned before upper structures are placed. Otherwise, epithelial rugae occur around the upper structure, making the provision of a healthy implant environment and hygiene would become impossible. Although upper structures longer than 4mm are available, usage of those will negatively affect loads over implants. The healing process of the mastoid region takes 3-4 months after those operations, while nasal, orbital, and mid-facial defects and radiotherapy-treated cases require at least 6 months [22, 28, 29, 32-34, 37, 40, 43, 49].

Implants Used in Maxillofacial Prosthetic Treatments

1. Intra-oral Implants
2. Extra-oral Implants

3. Zygomatic Implants

Implant contraindications

- Patients treated with high doses of radiotherapy,
- Patients with blood diseases,
- Patients with major psychological disorders,
- Patients with high risk of heart diseases,
- Patients with uncontrollable systemic diseases,
- Patients with alcohol and drug addictions,
- Young patients in adolescence,

Relative situations are as follows:

- Inadequate bone volume and bad bone quality,
- Hard and soft tissue pathologies,
- Patients who previously had addictions for tobacco, alcohol, and other substances.

Implant systems used in the maxillofacial area provide reinforcement in two ways:

1. Bar systems: bar systems are systems which function by locking on a bar attaching metal or plastic retentive clips over implants. Although retentive clips provide more retention than magnets, they have a greater tendency to corrode. When they are exposed to bodily fluids, they do not corrode, unlike magnets. Retentive clips are used for people who are able to use their hands efficiently, when the highest retention is desired for low muscle power regions. For example, bar systems are the systems which are most preferred for retention in auricular prosthesis.
2. Magnet systems: the other type of retention method is the usage of on-implant reinforcements which do not require upper structure preparation and which are not attached to each other. This technique is a method which only a maxillofacial prosthesis expert experienced in dental technology can handle. It was seen that detached reinforcement structures can be cleaned more efficiently by patients than patients can clean the more complicated upper structures [1, 2, 5, 17, 27, 29, 37, 40, 48, 53]

In recent years, samarium-cobalt and neodymium-ferrus-boron magnets, which are more durable than chrome-steel, are being produced in 3mm diameter form [4]. But magnet systems lose their retention specifications in time, which is why they need to be changed.

Usage of magnet systems in prosthesis retention is useful, especially for patients who are not able to use their hands to insert or extract prostheses.

INTRA-ORAL IMPLANTS

Principles of Implantation for Intra-oral Defects

A classic prosthesis applies excessive pressure on auxiliary teeth in these kinds of defects, which causes periodontal damages. Especially for large and one-sided defects, cross arch stabilization and resistance against vertical movement of prostheses are lost. As a result of this, teeth which play a key role in handling may be lost. In order to prevent that loss, a couple of implants which are placed in or around the defect region can decrease the load on auxiliary teeth, and they can provide cross arch stabilization and also effective resistance against forces changing their locations. Implants provide advanced osseo-integration with bony grafts. After grafts extracted from the iliac crest are placed in the zygomatic arc region and grafts extracted from the skull are placed on infra-orbital region, contra arc stabilization can be provided by a placement implant.

Principles of Implant Placements for Sub-Maxilla Defects

The mandible may be resected marginally or segmentally in the case of the tongue, extra-molar region of mouth bottom, and corpus tumors events. In the case of marginal defected maxilla, prostheses meeting functional needs can be effectively produced by placement many implants without applying grafts. For segmental defects, asymmetry and malocclusion due to inner down deviation of rear sub-maxilla segments can be removed by placing bone grafts extracted from the fibula or iliac crest on the defect region. With reinforcements of many implants placed on and around the defected region, a reasonably functioning prosthesis can be produced. A waiting time period for 3-9 months is required for the total binding of grafts on the host surface. It is also possible to transport osseo-integrated implants, which are placed on iliac bone or fibula before graft application, to the defect region together with grafts. Possible residual mini plates inside of the bones must be removed before implantation. If the mucosa covering the bone is too thick for attachment of trans-mucosal abutments, they must be thinned. For the planning phase before the implantation process, the dentition status of the antagonist arc and vertical dimension, the patient's ability to provide daily oral hygiene and the prosthesis' daily insertion and extraction properly must be considered, in addition to the construction level of surgery scar tissue, volume, position, innervations, and mobility of the residual tongue.

EXTRA-ORAL IMPLANTS

General Principles of Implant Supported Restorations of Extra-oral Defects

- Implant abutments must be as optimal as the covering skin can provide,
- For preventing destructive forces, subcutaneous skin layers should be thinned surgically, and this process must be performed 10mm away from abutments,
- Implants should be 1cm away from each other for hygienic purposes,
- Bars fixed between abutments must be in accordance with natural contours of the face and they must be designed in order to provide required hygiene needs,
- Implants must be placed at least 7mm away from hairy skin. If that is not possible, a skin graft must be applied.

PRINCIPLES OF IMPLANT IMPLEMENTATIONS FOR RESTORATIONS OF EXTRA-ORAL DEFECTS

Auricular Prostheses

Auricular defects constitute 70% of all maxillofacial defects. Surgical reconstruction of the auricular helix requires a surgery series taking a couple of years. An obtained auricular helix may not appear original and may not create a symmetrical face appearance. Transcutaneous implant usage is seen as an effective treatment option for auricular prostheses. By using this technique, it is possible to fabricate prostheses which are similar to anatomical structures and do not create trauma in the nearby tissues. These prostheses include retentive mechanisms.

The position of implants on the temporal region is very important for the aesthetic of auricular prostheses. Implants should be placed at the anti-helix level because retention systems need to be placed inside of the borders of auricular prostheses. Two pieces of implants placed in the temporal region can provide the retention of auricular prostheses. In such cases, two implants must be placed within 15mm away from each other and each of them must be 18mm away from the center of the auricular canal. One implant must be placed in the 9 o'clock position and the other in the 11 o'clock position for the right auricular, and one in the 1 o'clock position and the other in the 3 o'clock position for the left auricular (Figure 1). These traditional proposals should be accepted as a fixed principle. The exact positions of implants must be determined by producing a wax sample and using a surgical stent.

First of all, a wax model should be shaped for auricular prostheses in accordance with anatomical auricular specifications and then it will be placed such that it provides face symmetry. By using a wax auricular, a surgical stent can be produced from acrylic resin or vinyl acetate. When it is placed, the surgical stent must indicate the most appropriate regions to place the implants.

For auricular prostheses, generally two different retention systems are preferred and may be used alone or in combination.

For the first system, a gold base alloy bar is used in 2mm diameter form. This bar is soldered on a gold cylinder and then attached to implant abutments. The retention clips attaching the prosthesis to the bar are included in the prosthesis. The usage of the bar and clips system provides efficient prosthesis retention and force distribution. However, because the prosthesis includes a base part covering the bar, it is very difficult to reach the region beneath the bar and to clean it. Because retention is provided too effectively, insertion and extraction of the prosthesis may be difficult for patients who cannot use their hands effectively. In such cases, magnet auricular prostheses would be a better choice.

The second retention method is the magnet technique. The first method of this technique is to use a bar and magnets together. A bar structure attached to implant abutments is designed to create a seat for magnets. Magnets are placed into those seats by using acrylic resin. The other pair of magnets is placed into the silicone prosthesis. The magnets used in that system generally have a 6mm diameter and 2mm thickness. The bar-magnet system may create hygiene and aesthetic problems because they increase the volume of the structure which provides the retention [16, 29, 34, 37, 50].

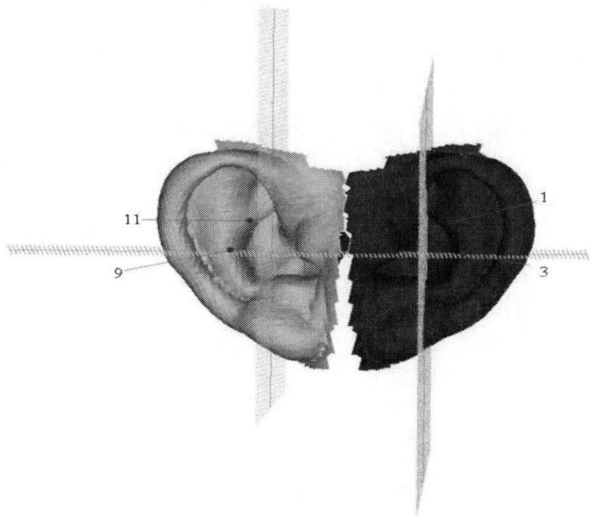

(This figure was prepared with IMTEC's ILUMA Vision Program).

Figure 1. Selecting the ideal implant sites on an auricular model.

The third alternative is to use a magnet system without using bars [4]. In this technique, magnets are directly attached to implant abutments. The main advantage of this technique is that it easily hides implant abutments inside of the borders of the prosthesis.

The previous periods of implant placement in auricular prosthesis has included the usage of four implants as reinforcement. Currently, it is accepted that two implants are enough to provide retention and reinforcement or auricular prostheses.

Nasal Prostheses

Nasal defects constitute 6% of all maxillofacial defect cases. The anterior nasal spine region beneath the nasal cavity has enough thickness to accommodate 3-6mm implants (Figure 2). The wax nasal model shaped before surgery may help in the determination of locations where implants will be placed and planning such that the holders will not affect the prosthetic contours [18, 32, 50]. In order to provide a stable surface for nasal prostheses, the defect region should be covered with a semi-thick skin graft. This process eliminates the destructive effects by decreasing the mobility of auxiliary tissues beneath the prosthesis. In order to increase stability, nasal prostheses should be extended through the lateral wall of the defect. For this purpose, anterior septal cartilage should be surgically lifted. To place one implant on each of two nasal eminence regions would provide enough retention. It is also recommended that abutments should be attached to each other with a bar and that bar must pass 15-20mm over the abutments.

Orbital Prostheses

Orbital defects constitute 20% of all cases. The problems which adhesives create in the temporal region are seen more frequently in the orbital region. Due to the adhesive coverage of orbital defect edges, consisted moisture causes inflammation in the soft tissues and it may therefore decrease the quality of life of the patient [33, 36, 40, 56].

Implant usage for the retention of orbital defects increases adhesive needs and prostheses became easier to use. They can be inserted and extracted without serious effort. This easy-to-use specification causes effective ventilation and protection of tissue health.

For the retention of an orbital prosthesis, bar and magnet systems are used. Generally, the bone, which has enough volume to place the implant in the orbita, exists in the lateral edge of the orbita. However, 3-4mm implants can be placed on bones at inferior, superior, and lateral regions of the orbita. Generally, three or four implants are required (Figure 3). The long axe of implants should traverse through the center of the orbita. The bar with a mono-block entrance way may not be achieved if some implants are heading in a posterior direction (cranial fossa) and some are heading in the reverse direction. If implants exist in both the upper and lower edges, generally, independent magnet systems are preferred. The wax sample of final prostheses must be used as a surgical stent in order to provide retention and an aesthetic improvement [25, 33].

The curved structure of the lateral wall of the orbita, the limited existence of bone, and limited accessibility of the region make restoration and implant protection more difficult. The circular positions of implants may make the production of a retention bar passively holding to all implant abutments more difficult. The bar also makes access to soft tissue around the implant abutments difficult. When magnet holders are used together with a bar, the accessibility problem of tissues is increased even more. The usage of magnets without a bar makes prosthetic processes easier and increases hygiene. Magnets help prostheses to find true positions during placement. Two or three implants are enough for retention of auricular prostheses.

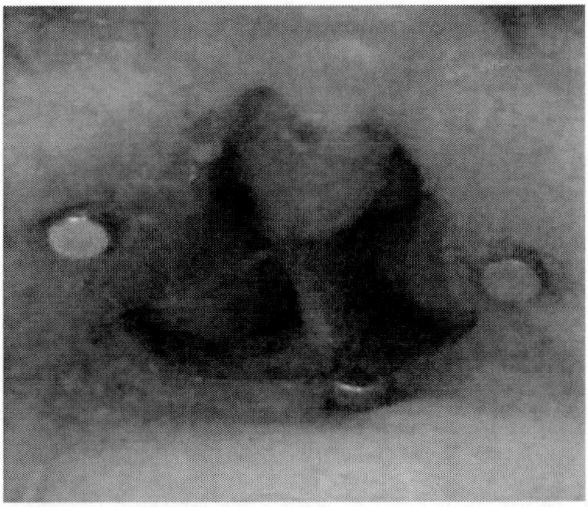

Figure 2. Using implants in nasal defects.

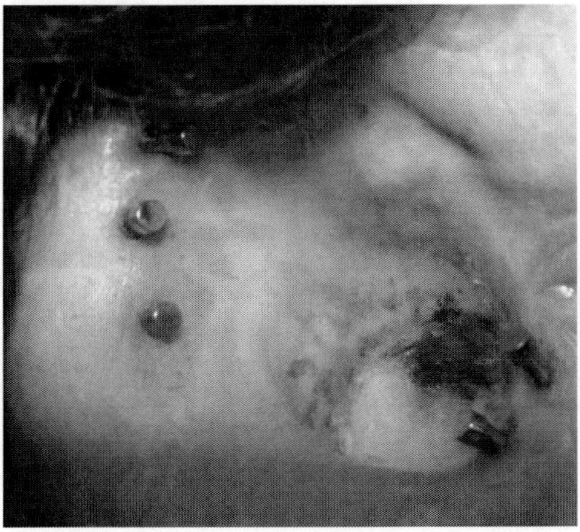

Figure 3. Using implants in orbital defects.

Ocular Implants

Ocular implants are materials placed into tissue sockets in order to make the production of prostheses easier. In 1960, Allen et al. [14] developed and embedded acrylic implant into canals for the passage of muscles for ocular prostheses. Then, by burrowing holes in acrylic Allen type implants rather than canals for the passage of muscles, the Iowa and Universal implants entered into usage. Today, most of the ocular prostheses are made of thermo-resistant, strong, light, and unbreakable acrylic materials.

If any material is not used in order to fill the empty space, there is a collapsed appearance because the size of the eye is restrained by a gap between the upper and lower eye lids. When the muscles move normally, the implant connected to ocular muscles also moves. So, the prosthesis gains movement ability and more realistic prostheses are obtained. For a growing child, the muscle function obtained by implementing an implant creates retention on orbital walls, providing the normal development of orbital growth.

Implant's Placement

Muscles are dissected from sclera after enucleation, where an implant is placed to control hemorrhaging, and ocular muscles are connected to the implant. Superior and inferior rectus muscles are sutured at 12 and 6 o'clock positions. After suturing the first two muscles, lateral and medial rectus muscles are sutured on the anterior surface of the implant at 3 and 9 o'clock positions. In order to prevent the implant from sinking into the eye socket base, inferior oblique muscles are sutured to superior rectus muscles. The suturing of the lateral rectus also decreases the ptosis. The plastic conformer is placed on the sutures and under the eye lid [9, 13, 38].

Implant Types

There are three basic ocular implant types:

An embedded implant is shaped like a sphere. The implant provides the movement for the prosthesis by moving the tissue bed where the prosthesis is placed.

A semi-embedded integrated implant is placed in a cone which is established by the ocular muscles. The frontal surface of the implant consists of a net system which is placed near the gap. Rectus muscles are connected to those nets. The eye prosthesis is made of male parts according to a gap in the implant. This improves the movement of the implant eye prosthesis, but generally is susceptible to infection and becomes lost is 2-5 years.

An embedded semi-integrated implant includes a body to which muscles are sutured or connected. When producing personal prostheses, an adverse contour is made on the back surface of the ocular prosthesis. There is always a tissue separating the artificial eye from the implant. So the movement opportunity can be protected, even if it is very limited. In fact, porous implants are made of an inorganic calcium phosphate salt, which is the main element of the human bone's inorganic matrix. Recently, bio-ceramic orbital implants have been developed in France (aluminum oxide, Alümina). It was approved by the FDA in America in 2002.

Research regarding ideal prostheses is still ongoing. The artificial eye was developed in order to provide a solution for people who lost their eyes in an accident or from a disease. But recently, researchers developed a robotic eye prosthesis which can perform all the duties of a real eye except seeing. The robotic eye is run by a small motor which shifts the eye ball according to the signals coming from the brain via electrodes at two sides of head.

Orbital implants are classified in different ways in terms of applied surgical technique, material type, shape, etc. According to standard surgical technique, they are classified into two main groups as integrated and non-integrated orbital implants. The non-integrated implants are placed inside the orbita, behind the tendon, and in the muscle cone. But there is no direct connection between muscles and the implant and they are generally spherically shaped. Integrated implants are directly connected with muscles. Also, those implants are classified into two groups as covered and non-covered implants. The covered implants are covered by a tendon and conjunctiva after the muscles are sutured. They may be shaped spherically or without any order. Some part of the implant is covered by different tissues, such as sclera, fascia lata, and dura mater, and then muscles are sutured to that tissue. Some implants have tunnels and sockets through which the muscles can be passed and then sutured. According to the material's structure, orbital implants are classified into two classes as solid (glass, acrylic, silicon, etc.) and porous. According to development order, porous implants are cattle spongiform bone, sea bream based hydroxyapatite, porous polyethylene, synthetic hydroxyapatite, and bio-ceramic [3, 5, 24, 36, 39, 46, 54, 56]

The hydroxyapatite (HA) ocular implant was first used by Perry [39]. In order to increase movement, Perry planned the usage of this material in 1983, while basic research studies were performed from 1983 until 1985. After enucleation and evisceration, HA implants were implemented to more than 80 patients from 1985 until 1989 in the scope of experimental protocol which is provided by the FDA. In 1989, the FDA approved the usage of HA as an orbital implant and released the usage.

Porous Orbital Implants

Porous implants are the most studied implants in recent years, and they are embedded and may be integrated to prostheses. They are, in fact, made from an inorganic calcium phosphate salt, which is the main element of human bone's inorganic matrix. HA has been used in reconstruction of orthopedic, maxillofacial, and maxillodental regions instead of bone. When it is used instead of bone, vascular elements and lamellae coalesce with bones and take place in reinforcement tissue. The aragonite (CaCo3, calcium carbonate) obtained from porites class bream can be transformed into calcium phosphate hydroxyapatite (Ca (PO4)6(OH2)) via a special hydrothermal reaction. The obtained material consists of ordered and mutually connected canals with a 500 micron diameter. They have many similarities with a bone's normal Havers system [46]. After the placement of that porous material into the orbita after enucleation and evisceration, it begins to be filled with fibro-vascular tissue. In approximately 4-6 months, the implant becomes filled almost completely in most of patients and it becomes a part of body. It is thought to minimize the infection development and risk of opening. Due to those specifications, the porous orbital implants showed advanced developments against the integrated implants which were used before.

Orbital Implant Size

The volume loss due to enucleation and evisceration is generally solved by allocating between prostheses and spheres which are implanted in the muscle conus.

Enucleation leads to a 25-30% loss in total volume of the orbita (6.5-7ml). The functions of orbital implants are to prevent retention of orbital tissues, to compensate for the volume loss caused by removing the eye, to reinforce the stability of prostheses, and to improve the mobility of prostheses. The volume of an eye ball is 7.2ml, but the volume of a prosthesis is approximately 2.5ml. For this reason, the volume of an orbital implant must be identical to the difference between the volume of the prosthesis (2.5ml) and the volume of the removed eye (7.2ml). If any implant with a smaller diameter than 21mm is used, the possibility of volume decrease in the orbita space is very high. In the beginning, the highest diameter which could be used was thought to be 18mm. People believed that if they used an implant larger than 18mm, the conjunctiva and tendon could be closed only by pressure, and so the implant could possibly be lost. For most adult patients, an implant with a 20-22mm diameter can be easily and without pressure placed into the tendon capsule and muscle conus. If any fatty atrophy, orbital soft tissue fibrosis, or retraction exists in the orbita or if any surgical operation is performed before enucleation, a larger implant is required [3, 6, 8, 9, 19, 21, 24, 25, 33, 36, 39, 44, 54].

There are several specifications which an ideal orbital implant must have:

1. The implant must be embedded totally,
2. It should be implemented easily,
3. It should be light-weight,
4. It should be smaller than a real glob and it should have enough volume for the prosthesis,
5. It should be able to be placed in muscle conus,
6. It should be inert and should not lead to any reaction,
7. Its structure should not allow any migration and exposition development,
8. It should not be resorbed over time,
9. Extra-ocular muscles must attach to the implant easily,
10. The prosthesis integration must be done completely for a complete transfer of movement.

The deep implant implementation into the muscle conus has some advantages:

- Larger implants may be used, and the enophthalmos and volume loss can be prevented,
- The risk of migration and exposition can be decreased,
- The tendon can be used for covering the implant as much as the anterior tendon capsule. So, the layer between the implant and conjunctiva can be reinforced. Porous implants are thought to fulfill most of those duties. The most important specifications of those implants are to be able to be vascularized and to be able to lead to appropriate results for integrating the prosthesis and implant;

- Because of vascularization, the infection risk is very low [10],
- The passage of fibro-vascular tissue through implant pores decreases the migration and exposition risk,
- Most of the weight of the prosthesis is carried by the implant via a pin. So, the weight is taken from the bottom eye lid, and the risk to the bottom eye lid and fornix ptosis decreases. The pulverization starts a few weeks after porous orbital implants are implemented into the tendon space after enucleation or into the sclera pouch after evisceration, but the complete vascularization requires at least 4-6 months [6, 38, 47]. After the end of this period, the completely mobile prosthesis can be achieved via pin implantation.

In order to visualize the vascularization, many different methods are used, including bone scintigraphy, Magnetic Resonance (MR), Ultrasound, and Colored Doppler. In Tec99m bone scintigraphy, Methylene Di-phosphate (MDP) is used as radio-nuclide material. Through an unknown mechanism, Tec99m showed that MDP accumulates at immature collagen of bone minerals. After implementing MDP intravenously, the visualization is performed in each of two lateral positions in 2-2.5 hours. MDP is stored in implant in proportion to vascularization. The MR contrasted with Gadolinium-DTPA is used in the other method. A 20ml contrast material is applied intravenously for more than 2 minutes; MR is started in 5 minutes. Some advantages of MR over against bone scintigraphy include the following:

- MR is a more sensitive and reliable method,
- MR provides 3D imaging and, thereby, more detailed information is available,
- The patient is not exposed to radioactive material by using MR, so its application is healthier,
- We can get information about qualification of vascularization via MR.

Because the sectioning is available via MR, the whole sphere can be evaluated. Normally, vascularization starts at the periphery and continues through the center. With MR, this separation can be made, and both vascularized and non-vascularized parts can be determined.

But because the counting is made from abroad, the vascularization in the periphery may mask the space in the center and false results may be obtained. Besides all those advantages, the biggest disadvantage of MR is that its price is higher than that of other methods.

The vascularization of porous orbital implants is required for covering the base and fornix with a hole which is obtained by screwing the conjunctival epithelium. This epithelium protects the implant from outer effects, particularly form infection. The epithelization of the hole which is opened after the screwing process and after successful blood builds up is finished in 4-6 weeks.

When the porous orbital implant is placed into the orbita, it leads to a minimally inflammatory reaction which is both non-allergenic and non-toxic. Reactions with giant cells are seen infrequently; it is reported in this reaction that the giant cells on the outer surface of the implant which keeps company with soft tissues shows osteoclastic activity [7, 13].

Implant Complication

1. **Ejaculating:** this is the most significant complication. An excessively large implant, implant material, the non-wirewound implantation after enucleation, the saturation of the tendon and conjunctiva under tension, infection, and the usage of non-appropriate prostheses in sockets are factors which contribute to the ejaculation. The ejaculation risk in porous implants is very low. The treatment is a secondary implantation, and the implants which are covered with autogenetic winding material are preferred. Also, a fatty skin graft should be preferred if the contradiction is associated with the case.
2. **Exposition**: the exposition of an implant started to be seen more frequently after the wide usage of especially porous implants. Exposition generally results with ejaculation in solid implants, but in porous implants with vascular reinforcement, it becomes a serious problem. The more biologically compliant materials of implants and the developments on techniques which are used in surgery have decreased the frequency, but they could not eliminate it completely. It is available to decrease the frequency by using implants of appropriate size, establishing a strong barrier at the frontal surface, suturing the scleral flaps in front of the implant as layers in evisceration, using the autologous and homolog winding material during enucleation, appropriately closing the tendon and conjunctiva layers, and preventing excessive pressures by applying place holders and prostheses.

3. **The migration of an implant:** migration is generally seen as downward migration of implant in orbita gravity, and it is most seen in non-integrated solid implants. The wound implantation decreases the frequency of migration. It is seen rarely in porous implants. Unless there is an apparent deformation in the socket and it prevents the implementation of prostheses, there is no need for treatment. The more complicated situations may lead to considerations regarding implant reposition or changing.
4. **The complications in porous implants regarding pins**: besides their contributions to the improvement of socket rehabilitation, porous orbital implants lead to some specific complications. The complications regarding pins are the most important ones. Infection, exposition, and migration are major complications. Minor complications are inflexion, formation of pyogenic granuloma, excessive secretion, bleeding, pin loss, and coverage.
   The main complications of porous orbital implants are as follows:
   - Exposition,
   - Migration,
   - Infection,
   - Ejaculation,
   - Pyogenic granuloma,
   - Mass formation,
   - Autonomous movement,
   - Pain,
   - Deficient implant blood build-up,
   - Complications involving a pin: ejaculation, inflexion, embedding.

By way of fibro-vascular tissue moving into its canals, porous orbital implants become a living part of the body, so the complications are expected at low rates. Buettner and Bartley [6] reported the exposition complications have a rate of 22%. Evidently, the exposition is the most common and most discussed complication in porous orbital implants. Their frequencies vary between 0 and 22% in different series.

The ejaculation risk in porous orbital implants is very low, while the presence of vascularized tissues under the implant smooth the treatment of that exposition through grafting. If the exposition occurs early after implantation, one must consider the deficient wound healing. For late occurring expositions, one must take into account the inappropriate relationship of prostheses and implants and the formation of necrosis due to excessive pressure, deficient coverage of tendon capsule over the implant, and deficient blood build-up in the implant. When we consider the complications according to types of porous orbital implants, there are serious differences between them in the literature. In a study conducted by Jordan et al., where they used four types of porous implants in 86 patients, they reported three natural HA, two bio-ceramic and one synthetic HA implant for exposition complications (7.7%). But then the authors expressed that they preferred to use the bio-ceramic orbital implants because of their bio-compliance, uniform porosity, and smoother surface [19, 22, 23, 24, 31, 39, 41, 46, 52, 55-56].

The implant infection is a rarely seen, but is a very serious complication. It may occur early (before prosthesis integration) or late (after integration). The early infections are due to deficient body resistance, vascularization problems around soft tissues, and implant expositions. For late developing infections, lesioned conjunctival mucosa is thought to be a reason for infection. Four possible mechanisms were reported for microorganism entrance: the period of placement of orbital implant, invasion style from exposition region, the process of screwing the implant for the pin, or the hematogenous dissemination during bacteremia. In the research literature, the implant infections have been reported in a frequency between 0.01% and 3.9% in different case presentations or patient groups [20, 22, 23].

The systemic or topical anti-biotic treatment with a wide spectrum creates good results in implant infections and implants rarely need to be displaced. The implant infection must be considered for patients with persistent conjunctiva inflammation, secretion, and implant exposition.

Combined Defect Prosthesis

Combined defects constitute 2% of all defects. For a determination of appropriate implantation areas in the maxilla, nasal, and orbital regions, a guide wax prosthesis model should be created. By using panoramic radiography and computerized tomography, the thickness and density of bone structures should be determined. It is possible to place implants in the glabella region of the frontal bone, beneath zygomatic arc, on pterygoid bone, at upper and lower orbital edges, and in alveolar processes. Bone grafts must be placed where the bone reinforcement is not sufficient. Large limited combined defect placement on bony structures on the periphery is more appropriate for their resistance to loads from their long axes. Implants placed at the center of defects transfer destructive forces to bones to which they are attached by being exposed to Class I level forces during rotational movements of the prosthesis [27, 37, 53, 55]. Trans-mucosal and trans-cutaneous implants can be used as combined implants in cases where intra- and extra-oral defects exist simultaneously.

Zygomatic Implants

In order to reinforce implants in maxillofacial region defects, zygomatic bones are used as well. Zygomatic implants are designed to be placed in those regions. Zygomatic implants have been developed in order to provide reinforcement for regions farthest from defect areas, and they have been used where general health conditions are not appropriate for surgery, such as when the reconstruction of large maxilla defects by using bone transplantation is not allowed by the patient. The length of implants placed on zygoma vary between 25mm and 60mm. for the success of these kinds of implants, at least two implants should be placed for each of right and left zygomatic bone regions, and then a cross arc stabilization should be provided by using rigid a structure made of bars. By using that design, chewing forces may be distributed through the long axes of implants [26, 28, 34, 37, 43, 48].

Magnets' Indications of the Retention of Implant Reinforced Facial Prostheses

a. Where there is muscle mobility near prosthesis:
   The prosthesis removed by muscle forces will be able to return to its original position due to magnetic power of magnets.
b. For patients who are not able to use their hands efficiently:
   It is easier to relocate a prosthesis to its original position with a prosthesis with magnet retention than that a prosthesis with clip retention.
c. In cases where the bone is thin and the force applied over the bone through the implant needs to be increased:
   Orbital defects are good examples of such kinds of clinical situations. Magnet prostheses can be removed by applying less power than that of clipped prostheses.

The mechanical principles governing implant reinforced crown-bridge prostheses are also valid for implant reinforced facial prostheses. A higher number of abutments and a larger surface decrease the force on each of abutment. Surface area, power, and stress concepts must be considered for implant reinforced facial prostheses [4, 29, 30, 37, 40, 43, 45].

Treatment Planning for Implant Reinforced Facial Prostheses

Surgery on malignant tumors in the head-neck region generally causes large tissue defects. Maxillofacial prostheses appear as an alternative for cases where surgical reconstruction cannot be applied. In previous periods, retention of the maxillofacial prosthesis has been generally made by using liquid- or spray-formed adhesives, adhesive bands, eyeglass connection, and hard or soft tissue retardations. Osseo-integrated implants used in treatment of edentulous cases are used for reinforcing facial prostheses and providing retention and stability.

The success of rehabilitation of patients with maxillofacial defects depends on patient's motivation, inter-disciplinary co-operation, and application of adequate surgical and prosthodontic techniques. Ideally, all the treatment options, such as surgical reconstruction and implant reinforced reconstruction, must be discussed before the surgical operation. If the organ to be removed by surgical operation is thought to be rehabilitated by implant reinforced prosthesis, soft and hard tissues around the surgical area should be prepared for placing implants by performing some arrangement during surgery. Bone regions which are important for the placement of osseo-integrated implants must be protected as much as possible or they must be resized to appropriate sizes to place implants by reconstructive processes. Thickness and mobility of the tissues near the defect edges are especially important for achieving aesthetic results. Because of muscle movements on the face, appearances of facial prostheses around areas where tissues move create aesthetic problems. Therefore, ideal indications of implant reinforced prostheses are the prosthetic treatment of resection in auricular, nasal, and orbital cases. In order to prevent inflammatory reactions, thin and hairless tissue must be created around the implant.

Because of defect size and position, existing bone volume and quality, soft tissue thickness and mobility differ individually in maxillofacial prosthesis implementation, making the general rules of maxillofacial prosthesis production for intra-oral rehabilitation very hard.

Depending on this, the number and location of implants to be placed will vary. While, generally, two implants are sufficient for the retention of auricular prostheses, as many implants as possible should be preferred in order to provide force distribution for medium-large maxillofacial defects. Maxillofacial defect treatment must be handled individually, and implants must be placed on appropriate positions with enough bone volume. In order to measure easier, implants should be placed in a parallel fashion. The extension of prosthesis borders increases the reinforcement and retention of the prosthesis. Preferably, the edges of the prosthesis should extend to tissues with less mobility.

Generally, the temporal bone, supra-orbital edge, lateral orbital edge, zygoma, piriform bump, and pterygoid process are accepted as anatomical regions having enough bone volume to reinforce implants.

Details of Regions in Implantation and Success

Although inflammatory reactions may occur around maxillofacial implants, they are successful in auricular, orbital, and nasal prosthesis reinforcement and they can have a success rate even in the treatment of toothless mouths by using standard implants.

Due to certain anatomical structures, we can find that implant success rates in implant reinforced maxillofacial prostheses could reach 95% and more in the mastoid region, 35-91% in the orbital region and 71-81% in the nasal region.

We can express the causes of lower success rates of implants in orbital region as follows:

- Patient cannot see the prosthesis region and so he cannot provide adequate hygiene,
- Older patients are not be able to use their hands effectively in such a way as to provide hygiene,
- Because the periosteal bone near the orbita is thin and atrophic, its remodelization specification is not adequate,
- Chronic inflammation around implant environment,
- Bone correction operations during surgery for making maxillofacial implants cover the bone.

The positioning and angling of an implant is a hardness belonging to a region and it is most frequently seen in orbital and mid-face prostheses.

Thinning the implant's environment decreases these complications. In case of trauma or tumor resection defects, skin and tissues under the skin are generally thin, and tissues are attached to the periosteum under them. This creates the ideal environment for protrusive implants. In the contrary scenario, there are thick and mobile tissues in cases of patients with congenital malfunctions. The soft tissue complications of those patients can be minimized by carefully thinning the flap in a second phase surgery or by placing skin grafts on implant regions as split thickness.

In most of the data, success rates for the auricular region in craniofacial implant placement exceed 95% and very few complications have been observed. Auricular implants can be placed on the mastoid region where it is determined to be the best location for implants in terms of bone volume and blood build-up. An angled incision is made 30mm behind the external auditory canal in the mastoid region. Typically, two implants are placed 15mm and 18mm behind the external auditory canal. The aim of this is to place a holder tissue bar beneath the anti-helix part of the prosthesis. Generally, two implants are enough for retention of an auricular prosthesis. If any hearing device will be used, or if there is any doubt about the success of existing implants, an additional implant can be placed. A non-tensioned periosteum with thinned environment is left and sewed around the implants. All of the subcutaneous fat, muscle, and collagen tissues are removed.

The success rate in nasal regions is between 85 and 90%. Very few soft tissue complications are observed for implants placed on the bottom of the nose. If the patient has no teeth in his maxilla, bone volume may be sufficient to vertically place implants on the nasal base. Two pieces of 4mm implants or longer dental implants can be placed in that region. If the teeth have roots, the lateral wall of the piriform aperture may be selected in order to place an implant horizontally. If nasal bones are resected, implants may be placed also on the glabella region. The second phase procedure for the nasal region is similar. In order to make immobile tissue layers with the use of upper structures as short as possible, tissue volume should be decreased as much as possible. Implants should be placed 8mm or 10mm away from the nasal base, and they should be placed in the anterior region so that the implants can be outside the attached and immobile tissues. If the implants are out of mobile tissues of lips, the incidence of soft tissue reaction around the implants increases. If implants are placed too far back, providing hygiene becomes harder.

The success rate of implants in the frontal bone and around the orbital is very low if those regions have been treated with radiation. Their failure rate is higher when compared with auricular and nasal base regions. Superior and lateral orbital edges are suitable for orbital defects. The usage of free skin grafts is not necessary for the orbital edge region. If the bone volume is sufficient, 4mm length implants are used. The usage of three implants to hold orbital prostheses is the best, but the risk of implant loss and high possibility of having radiotherapy in that region require the usage of more implants. For most cases, four or five implants are preferred. By placing those implants, the optimal positioning and angling must be considered. This is important, especially in order to avoid problems during insertion and extraction of the prosthesis. Also, for hygiene, there must be at least a 10-12mm distance between implants. The upper structure and the implants which do not affect contours of the orbital prosthesis must be considered and implants should not be placed too far in front.

Maxillofacial implants have a higher failure rate when compared with dental implants. This failure rate especially depends on the specific anatomical region where they are placed. Especially after resection, having enough bone volume may not always be found. A patient's ability to insert and extract the prosthesis, his ability to clean the tissue around implant, and the necessity of implants being in the borders of the prosthesis to be placed may create problems regarding the implant implementation when combined with limitations in bone volume. Most maxillofacial defects occur as a result of cancer surgeries, and, generally, radiotherapy assistance is needed after resection in those cases. This affects the short and long term success of craniofacial implant implementation. In his study, Nishimura determined the success rate of implants implemented in supra-orbital edges after radiation as 33%.

Functional loading factors are important factors for the long term success of implants. The transfer of force coming from implants to hard tissues creates a warning as remodeling or modeling. If the tensions around the implant exceed physiologic limits, the relation of the interface of bone and/or bone implant and the implant would be inevitably lost. For preparation of a comfortable upper structure and the ability of patient to clean the implant region, the distance between implants should be at least 10mm. Because of inadequate bone volume, implants cannot be placed in locations with equal distances and appropriate positions. This can cause problems in the preparation of upper structures and prostheses [1, 12, 17, 22, 27, 33, 43, 48-51, 53, 55].

We can summarize the factors which affect the success or failure of maxillofacial implants:

a. Bone volume and quality: this relationship is directly proportional. The dimensions of implants to be placed in bones must be determined in accordance with existing bone volume. When bone volume increases, longer and wider implants can be placed. As a result of studies, it is recommended that 3mm length implants should not be used.
   The inadequacy of compact bone may cause failure of implants by causing lack of primer stability. The mastoid process is a bone region of the facial skull where the bone quality and volume is good and adequate. There are dense compact bones in the edges of orbita and it affects stability in positive way. However, the volume of orbital edges is limited. Because most of the bones consist of compact bone, the lack of blood build-up and nutrition negatively affect implant success. Because the nasal bottom consists of loose trabecular bone, it negatively affects primer stability.
b. Hygiene: the tissue fluids in defect regions may accumulate and create dermatitis. That accumulation is seen most frequently in eye prostheses because there is a low possibility of a patient seeing the region with his single eye and to provide hygiene. The accessibility of the region is important and necessary for a patient's motivation and hygiene. Dermatitis may cause implant losses in upcoming periods. The handcraft and motivation of the patient is very important for providing adequate hygiene.
c. Radiation therapy: the effect of radiotherapy on implant success must be discussed. The dose of radiation, the implementation of hyperbaric oxygen treatment, the duration between radiotherapy and implant surgery, prosthetic design, and soft tissue status are important.

REFERENCES

[1] Asar, N. V., Yazıcıoğlu, H., Yaluğ, S. & Yılmaz, C. (2008). Implant supported facial prostheses. *J of Gazi University Faculty of Dentistry*, *25*, 41-49.

[2] Arcuri, M. R. & Rubenstein, J. T. (1998). Facial Implants. *Dent Clin North Am*, *42*, 161-175.

[3] Arora, V., Weeks, M., Halperin, E. C. & Dutton, J. J. (1992). Influence of corraline hydroxyapatite used as an ocular implant on the dose distribution of external beam photon radiation therapy. *Ophthalmology, 99*, 380.

[4] Atkins, A. D. & Roper-Hall, M. J. (1983). Magnetic orbital implants. *Br J Ophtalmol, 67*, 315-316 .

[5] Beumer, J., Curlis, J. A. & Firteil, D. N. (1979). Maxillofacial Rehabilitation: Prosthodontic and Surgical Considerations. St.Louis: The C.V. Mosby Company.

[6] Buettner, H. & Bartley, G. B. (1992). Tissue breakdown and exposure associated with orbital hydroxyapatite implants. *Am J Ophthalmol, 113*, 669 –73.

[7] Cheng, A. C., Wee, A. G., Li, J. T. & Archibald, D. (2002). A new prosthodontic approach for craniofacial implant-retined maxillofacial prostheses. *J of Prosthet Dent, 88*, 224-228.

[8] Danz, W. Sr. (1990). Mobility implants: A review. Adv. *Ophthalmic Plast Reconstr Surg, 8*, 46-52.

[9] Dutton, J. J. (1990). *Coroline hydroxyapatite as an ocular implant Ophthalmology, 3*, 371- 98.

[10] Ferrone, P. J. & Dutton, J. J. (1992). Rate of vascularization of corraline hydroxyapatite ocular implants. *Ophthalmology, 99*, 376-9.

[11] Flood, T. R. & Russell, K. (1998). Reconstruction of nasal defects with implant retained nasal prostheses. *Br J Oral Maxillofac Surg, 36*, 341-345.

[12] Gitto, C. A., Plata, W. G. & Schaaf, N. G. (1994). Evaluation of the peri implant epithelial tissue of percutaneous implant abutments supporting maxillofacial prostheses. *Int J Oral Maxillofac Impl, 9*, 197-206.

[13] Hornblass, A., Biesman, B. S. & Eviatar, J. A. (1995). Current techniques of enucleation: a survey of 5439 intraorbital implants and a review of the literature. *Ophthalmol. Plast Reconstr Surg, 11*, 77-86.

[14] Hughes, M. O., Jou, E. M. & Young, S. R. (2006). Lee Allen, Ocularist. *J of Ophtalmic Prosthetics*, 13-25.

[15] Ismail, J. Y. H. & Zaki, H. S. (1990). Osseointegration in maxillofacial prosthetics. *Dent Clin North Am, 34*, 327-341.

[16] Jacobsson, M., Tjellström, A., Fine, L. & Jansson, K. (1992). An evaluation of auricular prostheses using osseointegrated implants. *Clinical Otolaryngology & Allied Sciences, 17*, 482-486.

[17] Jacobsson, M., Tjellstrom, A., Fine, L. & Anderson, H. (1992). A retrospective study of osseointegrated skin-penetrating titanium fixtures

used for retaining facial prostheses. *Int J Oral Maxillofac Implants*, *7*, 523-528.

[18] Jensen, O. T., Brownd, C. & Blacker, J. (1992). Nasofacial Prostheses Supported by Osseointegrated Implants. *Int J Oral Maxillofac Implants*, *7*, 203-211.

[19] Jordan, D. R. (2004). Problems after eviseration surgery with porous orbital implants. Experience with 86 patients. *Ophthal Plast Reconst Surg*, *20*, 374-380.

[20] Jordan, D. R., Brownstein, S. & Faraji, H. (2004). Clinicopathologic analysis of 15 explanted hydroxyapatite implants. *Ophthal Plast Reconstr Surg*, *20*, 285-90.

[21] Jordan, D. R., Gilberg, S. & Bawazeer, A. (2004). Coralline hydroxyapatite orbital implant (Bio-Eye): Experience with 158 Patients. *Ophthal Plast Reconst Surg*, *20*, 69-74.

[22] Karakoca, S., Aydin, C., Yılmaz, H. & Bal, B. T. (2010). Retrospective study of treatment outcomes with implant-retained extraoral prostheses: survival rates and prosthetic complications. *J of Prosthet Dent*, *103*, 118-26.

[23] Kaltreider, A. S. & Newman, A. S. (1996). Prevention and management of complications associated with the hydroxyapatite implant. *Ophthal Plastic and Recontsr Surg*, *12*, 18-31.

[24] Kazim, M., Katowitz, J. A., Fallon, M. & Piest, K. L. (1992). Evaluation of a collagen hydroxyapatite implant for orbital reconstructive surgery. *Ophthal PlastReconstr Surg*, *82*, 94-108.

[25] Kovacs, A. F. (2000). A follow-up study of orbital prostheses supported by dental implants. *Int J Oral Maxillofac Implants*, *58*, 19-23.

[26] Landes, C. A. (2005). Zygoma implant-supported midfacial prosthetic rehabilitation:a 4-year follow-up study including assessment of quality of life. *Clin Oral Impl Res*, *16*, 313-325.

[27] Leonardi, A., Buonaccorsi, S., Pellacchia, V., Moricca, L. M., Indrizzi, E. & Fini, G. (2008). Maxillofacial prosthetic rehabilitation using extraoral implants. *J Craniofac Surg*, *19*, 398- 405.

[28] Malavez, C., Abarca, M., Durdu, F. & Daelemans, P. (2004). Clinical outcome of 103 consecutive zygomatic implants: a 6–48 months follow-up study. *Clin Oral Impl Res*, *15*, 18-22.

[29] McKinstry, R. E. (1979). *Fundamentals of Facial Prosthetics.* Arlington; ABI Professional Publications: 1995. Muğan, N. Maxillofacial Prostheses. Istanbul: Gençlik Press.

[30] Mules, P. H. (1885). Evisceration of the globe with artificial vitreus. *Trans. Ophthalmol. Soc. U.K.*, *5*, 200-10.

[31] Nishimura, R. D., Roumanas, E., Moy, P. K. & Sugai, T. (1996). Nasal defects and osseointegrated implants: UCLA experience. *J Prosthet Dent*, *76*, 597-602.

[32] Nishimura, R. D., Roumanas, E., Moy, P. K., Sugai, T. & Freymiller, E. G. (1998). Osseointegrated implants and orbital defects: UCLA Experience. *J of Prosthet Dent*, *79*, 304-309.

[33] Nishimura, R. D., Roumanas, E., Sugai, T. & Moy, P. K. (1995). Auricular prostheses and osseointegrated implants: UCLA experience. *J of Prosthet Dent*, *76*, 553-558.

[34] O'Connell, J. E., Cotter. E. & Kearns, G. J. (2011). Maxillary reconstruction using zygomatic implants: a report of two cases. *J Ir Dent Assoc*, *57*, 146-55.

[35] Ow, R. K. K. & Amrith, S. (1997). Ocular prosthetics:Use of a tissue conditioner material to modify a stock ocular prosthesis, *J of Prosthet Dent*, *78*, 218-222.

[36] Parel, S. M., Branemark, P. I. & Tjellstrom, A. (1986). Osseointegration in maxillofacial prosthetics Part II: extraoral applications. *J Prosthet Dent*, *55*, 600-606.

[37] Parr, G. R., Goldman, B. M. & Rahn, A. O. (1983). Surgical considerations in the prosthetic treatment of ocular and orbital defects. *J Prosthet Dent*, *49*, 379-385.

[38] Perry, A. C. (1990). *Integrated orbital implants*. In: Bosniak SL, Smith BC, eds. Advances in Ophthalmic Plastic and Reconstructive Surgery. New York: Permagon Press;1990.

[39] Roumanas, E. D., Freymiller, E. G., Chang, T. L., Aghaloo, T. & Beumer III, J. (2002). Implant-retained prostheses for facial defects: an up to 14-year follow-up report on the survival rates of implants at UCLA. *Int J Prosthodont*, *15*, 325-322.

[40] Sarvananthan, N., Amanda, J. & Liddicoat, G. T. (1999). Synthetic hydroxyapatite orbital implants: a clinical and MRI evaluation. *Eye*, *13*, 205-8.

[41] Schneider, L. R. (1986). Modified ocular prosthesis impression technique. *J of Prosthet Dent*, *55*, 482-485.

[42] Schoen, P. J., Ragheobar, G. M., van Oort, R. P., Reintsema, H., van der Laan, B. F., Burlage, F. R., Roodenburg, J. L. & Vissink, A. (2001). Treatment outcome of bone-anchored craniofacial prostheses after tumor surgery. *Cancer*, *15*, 3045-50.

[43] Shields, C. L., Shields, J. A. & Potter, P. (1992). Hydroxyapatite orbital implant after enucleation. Experience with initial 100 consecutive cases. *Arch Ophthalmol*, *110*, 333-8.

[44] Shields, C. L., Shields, J. A., Eagle, R. C. & De Potter, P. (1991). Histopathologic evidence of fibrovascular ingrowth four weeks after placement of the hydroxyapatite orbital implant. *Am J Ophthalmol*, *111*, 363-66.

[45] Simsek, İ. B. (2005). *Porous orbital implant and complications*, Thesis, Istanbul: Istanbul Press.

[46] Su, G. W. & Yen, M. T. (2004). Current trends in managing the anophthalmic socket after primary enucleation and evisceration. *Ophthal Plast Reconstr Surg*, *20*, 274-80.

[47] Scolozzi, P. & Jaques, B. (2004). Treatment of Midfacial Defects Using Prostheses Supported by ITI Dental Implants. *Plast Reconstr Surg*, *114*, 1395-1404.

[48] Taylor, T. D. (2000). *Clinical Maxillofacial Prosthetics*. Illinois; Quintessence Publishing Co. Inc.

[49] Tjellström, A., Yontchev, E., Lindström, J. & Branemark, P. L. (1985). Five-years' experience with bone-anchored auricular prostheses. *Otolaryngol Head Neck Surg*, *93*, 366-372.

[50] Tolman, D. E. & Taylor, P. F. (1996). Bone-anchored craniofacial prosthesis study. *Int J Oral Maxillofac Impl*, *11*, 159-168.

[51] Van Blitterswijk, C. A., Hesseling, S. C., Grote, J. J., Koerten, H. K. & de Groot, K. (1990). The Biocompatability of hydroxyapatite ceramic. *J Biomed Mater Res*, *24*, 433- 42.

[52] Visser, A., Ragheobar, G. M., van Oort, R. P. & Vissink, A. (2007). Post-academic dental specialities 17. Implant-retained craniofacial prostheses. *Ned Tijdschr Tandheelkd*, *114*, 460-467.

[53] Wilson, M. W., Wobig, J. L. & Dailey, R. A. (1998). Infection of a porous polyethylene orbital implant with Capnocytophaga. *Ophthal Plast Reconstr Surg*, *14*, 398-402.

[54] Wolfaardt, J. F., Wilkes, G. H. & Anderson, J. D. (2000). *Craniofacial Osseointegration-Prosthodontic Treatment*. Illinois; Quintessence Publishing Co. Inc.

[55] You, J. R., Seo, J. H., Kim, Y. H. & Choi, W. C. (2003). Six cases of bacterial infection in porous orbital implants. *Jpn J Ophthalmol*, *47*, 512-8.

[56] Yazıcıoğlu, H. & Yafuğ, S.(1995). Custom ocular prosthetics. *J of Gazi Univercity Faculty of Dentistry*, *12*, 117-120.

Chapter V

COLOR CONCEPT AND COLORING IN MAXILLOFACIAL PROSTHESES

1. COLOR

Color is a sense which occurs in the brain as a result of light reflecting from materials and arriving in the eye. The visible light, consisting of various colors, has wavelengths ranging from 380 to 780 nanometers. Visible light exists as a short band in the electromagnetic wave spectrum, which includes X rays, gamma rays, ultraviolet rays, infrared radiation, and radio waves. This short band is able to be seen by the human ocular system. The human eye can see only waves with wavelengths between 380-780 nanometers on the electromagnetic spectrum. Seeing itself is a psychological and physiological case. Light causes a photo-chemical reaction on the eye's nerve layer, which is called the retina. Electrical signals results from those reactions and arrive to the seeing unit in the brain through optic nerves. By using information in the memory about seeing, the brain detects and interprets the new coming signals.

Because color is an electromagnetic light energy having a wavelength which the human eye can perceive, it has different wavelengths differing according to each item radiating light. If sunlight is refracted via a prism, the white light is divided into various colored lights having different wavelengths. Those colored lights are called a spectrum. A light spectrum consists of various colors, and to be visible, it is enough to have rays with 515, 480, and 650nm wavelengths, which create the senses of green, blue, and red colors.

The colored appearance of materials depends on the electromagnetic waves included by light and the structure of material. The colors of materials are determined according to their reflection, absorption, and glittering of the energy of the light dropping on them. Materials which seem red absorb the blue and yellow wavelengths of light rays. The other primary colors, yellow and blue, create the color of green by combining. The color of purple consists of combination of red and blue rays. Color tones differ due to different combinations of rays with different wavelengths. The material absorbing all the wavelengths of light appears as black. If the rays return without any absorption, white color appears. If the rays are absorbed equally by a material, the material seems gray. A material appearing to have a color under sunlight seems to be different under lamp light or candle light, like having different color tones. Because the light sources changed, the rays which they radiate change as well.

Color is the sense which is created by rays through visual sense. In other words, color is the effect which light leaves on us by being reflected from materials. The bright and alive sight of materials on sunny days and the loss of those appearances on overcast days show that color depends on light. When the sunlight is passed through a prism, seven different color groups arise. When those colors stored in sunlight come over a material, that material absorbs some part of those colors and it reflects some part of them. As a result of that reflection, materials appear as the color which they reflect to us. If the tips of color group in sunlight come together, a color circle arises.

The following principles are true regarding sight events:

- The incidence of the rays is **physical**,
- The processes arising as a result of those rays are **physiologic**,
- The perception of the material by the brain is **psychological**.

The wavelengths of rays creating different color senses are different. The ray with the lowest incidence angle is red and the ray with highest incidence angle is purple. Because the structures of light and paint are different, the color of black arises when all the paint colors are mixed in equal amounts and the color of white arises when all the light colors are mixed in equal amounts. The white and black colors arising as a result of combination of all colors are in fact colorlessness. Neither black nor white is considered a color, for they are neutral.

Light - Shadow: The concept which makes visible the volume and depth of materials is called light-shadow. Light sources are the sun, moon, and artificial light sources. A single light source cannot illuminate all sides of materials equally at a single time. The parts of the object nearest to the light source seem bright, while the parts farthest from the light source seem dark, and the parts between light and shadow seem to be the same color as the material. The degree of illumination of a material is called tone. When we evaluate the light and shadow status of materials enlightened by a light source, we observe four main situations.

1. **Light tone** (enlightened part): This is the brightest part, where light rays are steepest on a material. This part cannot give the actual color of material.
2. **Actual tone:** This is the part where light rays slope and there are no reflections or shining. This part gives the actual color of material. For round materials, this part is called the passage because light and dark sights conjugate there.
3. **Dark Tone** (own shadow): This is the darkest part of material where there is no light. Light – dark tones are the tone degrees when the color passes from light to shadow.
4. **Shadow:** This is the shadow of the material on the floor or ground. It reflects the shape of material. The enlightenment on the ground by reflection of the light on material is called a reflex.

   We should not forget that these three color factors determine the color of materials:

   a. **The material's own color (local color):** The own color of object-material,
   b. **The color differing due to light (tonal color):** The changed appearance of the color as a result of effects of light and shadow,
   c. **Reflecting Color:** The colors reflecting from other objects in the environment.

      Those factors affect these three additional factors:

   d. The color of light,
   e. The density of light,
   f. The atmosphere.

Main (primary) colors:

Red
Blue
Yellow

Intermediate Colors:

Green
Orange
Purple

Neutral colors:

White
Black
Grey

The intermediate color arising as a result of the combination of two main colors is the supplementary of the main color not attended into combination. Because they show the real powers of each other and stimulate each other, they are contrary colors at the same time.

Red - its supplementary - Green
Blue - its supplementary - Orange
Yellow - its supplementary - Purple

General classification of colors contrast / opposite colors

Yellow ------------------ Purple
Red ------------------ Green
Blue ------------------ Orange

Supplementary Colors

Purple ------------------ Blue
Red ------------------ Orange
Yellow ------------------ Green
Hot and Dark-hot: materials with those colors become prominent.
Cold and Light-cold: The materials with those colors remain in background.

Value: Value expresses a color's degree of lightness or darkness. There is a tone difference between dark blue and light blue. In a 10 grade tone scale showing grey tones from black to white, white is the brightest color and black is the darkest color. To change the value of a color is possible by adding black or white.

Density (saturation degree): This is the measurement of saturation quality or strength of a color. The saturation quality of the colors in the spectrum is in highest level.

Color Spectrum

Psychologic properties of colors: Fire's yellow-red color evokes the hot color and ice's blue-green color evokes cold color, and these evocations prompt the division of colors into two classes: hot colors and cold colors.

Hot colors: Red, yellow, orange

Cold colors: Green, purple, blue

The determination for intermediate colors of purple and green depends on combination of hot and cold colors in those colors. It is not possible to settle an exact delimitation.

Color is an element which is perceived visually, has much sensational efficiency and functions for aesthetic purposes.

According to structural properties of colors, their sensational effects are summarized as follows.

1. Color affects the environment where it is used. For example, while using bright colors in a room creates a cheerful and excited effect, using opaque colors creates relaxing effects.
2. Colors cause a place to gain unity and diversity. While similar colors, ordered in hot or cold colors, or an order consisting of only one color contributes to a sense of unity, an order consisting of different colors creates a sense of diversity.
3. It expresses the **own-property** of the material.
4. Color determines the form of the material. A single line, a surface with two dimensions, or a volume with three dimensions are determined with the usage of opposite colors.

5. Color affects ratios. The vertical usage of opposite colors stimulates one's sense of width, while the horizontal usage of opposite colors stimulates one's sense of height.
6. Color reveals the scale of an object. Determining the scale of a structure consisting of only one color is difficult, while determining the scale of a structure with opposite colors is easier when looking from far away.
7. Color creates a sense of weight. Dark colored elements seem heavier, while light colored elements seem lighter.

Just like many other elements, research regarding the nature of colors is very rich. The rich color harmonies in nature include much opposition. Colors gain value when they come together. Color relationships occur in frames of compliance or opposition. Color compliances constitute harmony. Generally effective, beautiful, and understandable harmonies rely on color oppositions. A color harmony in an order generally comes from the unity of opposite colors.

Newton, who succeeded in distinguishing the bands sunlight by using a prism, also found which colors are acquired by combining other colors. After Newton's theories established the study of color to be a branch of science, the sources of colors in our lives have been researched by using modern techniques, though Newton's theories have not been falsified.

Here are the combinations of colors:

Turquoise	blue + green + white
Purple	red + blue
Green	yellow + blue
Pink	red + white
Skin color	brown+ white+ dark red
Maroon	red+ black
Orange	yellow + red
Light pink	yellow+ black+ white
Grey	black+ white
Light green	turquoise + black
Light green	Blue + green + black+ white
Mold green	Blue + green + light black+ white
Brown	yellow+ black+ red
Brown	orange+ black
Brown	orange + purple
Brown	red + green

Tobacco	red + brown
Tone of tobacco	brown + red + yellow
Navy	red + dark blue
Gold	yellow + brown
Khaki green	brown + green
Olive green	Blue + light green
Oil green	yellow + light black
Light rose	purple + red
Light copper red	star+ brown + red
Smoke	lilac + purple
Lilac	Blue + red + light white

Details of Care by Coloring

Combination tip 1: Add the dark color to light color

A very small amount of darkness has the power to significantly change the light color, but the same is not true for the reverse. For this reason, do not add white to blue if you would like to create light blue. Instead, add blue to white.

Combination tip 2: Add opaque colors to transparent colors

When mixing transparent and opaque colors, add the opaque color slowly.

Combination tip 3: Prefer colors with a single pigment

In order to have very bright and dense mixtures, be careful that the colors you mix are made of only one pigment. The sterling brands express how many pigments exist in their tubes.

Combination tip 4: Perfect brown and grey mixtures

In order to find compliant grays and browns for your picture, do not use your unmixed supplementary colors. Start from existing colors in your pallet, such as red/green, yellow/purple, and blue/orange.

Combination tip 5: Do not mix for long time

Do not consider mixing long by mixing two colors. Do not touch the mixture after a couple of pushes. By doing this, you will see that colors will be more beautiful.

Light-Eye Relationship

The eye's starting point for vision is the retina, where light rays hit. There are two classes of nerves in the retina which are sensitive to brightness and color. The nerves sensitive to light strength are called rods and the nerves sensitive to color are called as cones. When the light strength is not adequate, cones do not work and color sense disappears. In those cases, sight is provided by rods, though the colors of visible materials are different tones of grey and black, according to their own colors. There are three kinds of cones which allow us to see colors. Cones which are sensitive to red (long wave) light are called L-cones, or red cones. Cones which are sensitive to green (medium wave) light are called M-cones, or green cones. Cones which are sensitive to blue (short wave) light are called S-cones, or blue cones. The different amounts of unique colored light coming in unison with other colors are seen as one color by uniting in those cones. When the red light and green light come to the eye together, the color perceived is yellow. So the eye cannot distinguish whether the coming yellow light is yellow-colored or a mixture of red and green. Color blindness results from the lack of one of those cones.

The effect of light mixtures on sight

When differently-proportioned mixtures of red, blue, and green light come to eye, they create the senses of all colors. For this reason, these three colors are accepted as primary colors. The mixtures of primary colors in equal amounts create intermediate colors. Those colors are yellow, cyan, and magenta. When the primary colors come to the eye in equal amounts, they create the sense of white. The colors which create the sense of white in the eye when they come together are called supplementary colors. The supplementary colors are red and cyan (greenish blue), green and magenta (reddish purple) and blue and yellow.

Light – Object Relationship

A material receiving light may reflect, absorb, or transmit the light. The item will be seen as the same color as the light which it reflects. Because no light come to the eye from materials which absorb the light, they appear black. So, black is not a color. The effect of black is to not be able to recognize the item.

The appearance of materials in different colors has different physical and chemical causes. One of those causes is the colorization of materials. Painted materials reflect the light or absorb some light colors. Accordingly, the light coming from a material by reflection is the light lacking certain wavelengths, and thus, certain colors. A yellow painted material reflects the yellow color when it is enlightened with primary light colors and it absorbs the blue and red colors. That combination stimulates yellow sense in eyes.

Because paint is not a light source, there is no mixture of light color and paint color. Because paints appear as the same color as those which they reflect, the colors constituted by paint mixtures are different from light mixtures. The primary colors in paint mixtures are yellow, magenta, and cyan.

If the three primary colors of paint would be mixed in equal amounts, yellow paint absorbs blue light, magenta paint absorbs green light, and cyan paint absorbs red light. So the main colors of light cannot reflect from that material and the material will appear as black color. If two primary colors of paint were to be mixed in equal amount, they only reflect the color which is common for the two.

If yellow and magenta paints are mixed in equal amounts, yellow paint absorbs blue light and magenta paint absorbs green light, so the material would appear red because red light is reflected from both of paints.

Most of materials around us are painted. The behavior of light on painted surfaces is a little bit complicated. The painted surface under sunlight reflects some of colors in light and absorbs other colors of light. The surface appears as the color of the most significant light coming from to lights to the eye.

The main colors of paints (yellow-magenta-cyan) each absorb only one main color of light. They reflect the other two main colors. They reflect the adjacent colors of primary light colors.

The primary colors of paints reflect all the colors of light (red-green-blue), whether strong or weak. The ones reflected strong are their own colors and ones reflected weak are their adjacent colors. When the light coming to the eye decreases (the decrease of light power), the effect of light on the color cones decreases. Rod cells then come into play and the eye perceives the light in grey tones.

Different lamps are used in houses, streets, or saloons. Some of these lamps spread all the colors of light and some of those lamps spread light in only one color. This is why the color of a dress which we loved under a particular lamp may seem different under sunlight.

The Color of Materials under Experimental Conditions

In order to simplify the cases, weak reflections from materials are not considered. Thereby, grey tones are considered as black color. Unless otherwise indicated, the color of light used for question purposes is assumed to be the primary light colors of the intermediate colors, which are mixtures of primary colors. White light is the light mixture where there are red, blue, and green lights. Because there is no red in pure yellow light, it can be said that it is reflected from red surfaces weakly. But if the light is not identified as pure, we can understand that it is a yellow light consisting of red and green lights. In that case, the surface enlightened with yellow light absorbs the color green and reflects the color red.

According to the color in which the materials seem under white light,

1. Non-transparent colors reflect the light of the same color as them strongly and the light of the adjacent color weakly.
2. Transparent colors transmit the light of same color as them strongly and the light of the adjacent color weakly.

Because the weak light cannot be recognized strongly by cone cells, eyes cannot efficiently see the colors. But rod cells are stimulated and the sight process is performed in grey tones. Because of that property, the lights in adjacent colors of materials are not considered. According to this, enlightened things appear with their own color, not transparently. They absorb other colors. If the object is transparent, it transmits its own color and absorbs other colors.

Colors are classified as chemical colors and light colors. The main colors used in pictures are blue, red, and yellow. However, the main light colors in pictures are red, blue, and green.

The main colors in light are red, blue and green.

Green+Red = Yellow
Green+Blue = Cyan
Blue+Red = Meganta

The main colors in painting are accepted as red, blue, and yellow [10, 15].

2. Colorization of Maxillofacial Prostheses

An important stage in the preparation of maxillofacial prostheses is colorization. For successful imitation of a patient's skin, the transparent primary material of prosthesis is colored through the use of various coloring agents. The defect region in the face is very important for providing aesthetic and masking prostheses in order to reflect the desired effects on the prosthesis [18, 19, 20].

When the colorization process of maxillofacial prostheses begins, the first stop is to determine the color of the region where the prosthesis will be placed. If the clinician can determine the main color of the facial region, he can achieve the true colorization by applying different effects according to defect location. Let us explain some important points of determining the main color. There are four necessary principles for providing natural colorization of maxillofacial prostheses: color, heterogeneity, translucency, and main structure.

Many factors play a role for true perception of color. Those factors are as follows:

a. The energy distribution of light,
b. Where the color is seen,
c. The propagation properties of materials in terms of absorption, reflection, and passage,
d. Sensitivity of eyes.

If the light is thought to be a transverse wave movement, it becomes easy to understand by measuring color. These three terms are used for explaining transverse wave movement:

1. Amplitude: the distance which light switches according to its transmittance environment.
2. Frequency: the number of cycles of the wave per second.
3. Wavelength: the distance between two waves.

3. Color Measurement Methods

The perception of the color of a material is the result of a physiological response to a physical stimulus. This is a subjective experience. All visible colors include only three basic colors; red, green, and blue. Other colors are acquired through appropriate mixtures of those main colors. For example, yellow is acquired through the appropriate mixture of green and red. Two basic methods are used for color measurement of prosthetic materials:

1. Instrumental methods,
2. Visual methods.

Instrumental methods include computerized color formulation, spectro-photometer, and calorimeter. Instrumental or visual methods are used for determination of color. The method mostly used in dentistry is visual color determination, which is applied in front of the patient by visually comparing the colors. But the usage of visual methods in choosing colors was deemed inadequate, which is an ongoing problem in dentistry. More scientific and consistent methods are needed for choosing colors for the purposes of restorative dentistry. Since they were introduced to dentistry, spectro-photometers and calorimeters have been used in research and could not be used in clinical stages.

Instrumental color analysis has many advantages against visual methods. Because the instrumental color determination is objective, the proportions can be accurately determined at a faster rate. Because there are differences between individuals in terms of color perception through visual methods, people understood that the visual method was not appropriate. Visual color perception depends on physiological and psychological responses of observers to radiant energy stimuli. Inconsistencies may depend on uncontrollable factors such as tiredness, age, senses, environmental lighting conditions, the position of light, and metamerism. Additionally, those factors stimulate different senses for different observers [2, 6, 9, 13, 14, 22].

Despite of all those limitations, human eyes can often recognize even minimal differences in colors. Their ability to determine the difference in terms of dimension and nature of color is limited. The instrumental measurement can determine the amount of color and transfer the data to other people correctly and uniformly. Development of more advanced calorimeters and spectro-photometers resulted in the increased usage in dental research. Calorimeters provide measurements in CIELAB units such as (L*, a*, b*) and those measurements can be used for comparisons of color parameters when they are analyzed mathematically. The usage of CIELAB calorimetric system is preferred for dental usages and there are some developments to this concept. The developments in optical electronic and computer technology give a larger usage area compared with calorimeter technique. Though important research has been conducted in this area, there is no specific instrument for usage in clinical dentistry yet [2, 15].

The achievement of visual compliance of maxillofacial prostheses and the human face has always been very difficult. But this compliance is very important for the success of this type of prosthesis. Maxillofacial silicones are colored in clinical implementations by using two different methods: intrinsic and extrinsic coloration. In some cases, the intrinsically colored silicone may be re-colorized extrinsically after elastomatic vulcanization. That colorization process is performed clinically. Until the natural tone of the skin of the patient is achieved, natural paints are slowly added into translucent silicone elastomers and then silicone elastomers are shaped into the desired form. In colorization sets prepared by various companies, all the colors of the rainbow exist. Besides those coloring agents, instruments such as colored yarn are used for achieving desired effects in related regions. Using colors in a color scale, coloring agents are clinically added into the main materials slowly until the desired color is acquired. The final color compliance depends on the clinician's color distinguishment ability and preferences [6, 9, 16, 17-21].

The preparation of maxillofacial prostheses to be compliant with skin color is required for an adequate aesthetic result, but it is very difficult to achieve. For this reason, the color of skin must be determined exactly.

The colorization of prostheses varies due to the various preferences of clinicians and the specific materials and methods used. There are various scales of skin tones for different materials. There are many kinds of colorant used in maxillofacial prostheses. Among the colorants are ceramics, enamel porcelain, water-based paints, cellulosic paints, photo paints, acrylic–resin paints, food colorants, pastels, oil-paints, natural pigments, and nylon fibrils [5, 7, 8, 11, 21].

The surface details and character of the face must be imitated through intrinsic and extrinsic colorization. Though techniques vary due to the timing and method of colorization of the prosthesis, natural colorization can be acquired through intrinsic coloring. Intrinsic coloring is preferred because it is stronger and it allows for the simulation of a labeled structure of skin. The permeability and depth of the skin can be acquired better through this colorization method. Intrinsic coloring has some functional advantages. Because it is affected very little by environmental conditions, it increases the usage life of prostheses and processed surface properties, which are generally lost in the process of extrinsic coloring.

Extrinsic coloring is the method which is applied on totally polymerized and unmolded prosthetic surfaces. Although it provides predictable results and it is performed by looking at directly the patient's skin color, this method is very environmentally- and usage-sensitive. The basic color of the prosthesis must be in accordance with the lightest color of the corresponding region tissues. If the basic color would be darker, more significant color differences will occur while applying extrinsic coloring for aesthetical compliance [19-21].

The coloring must be performed clinically and under appropriate lighting. Colors and tone differences must be evaluated under different light sources. The aesthetic result and color stability of prostheses are the most important factors in the clinical success of facial prostheses.

REFERENCES

[1] Andreopoulos, A. G. & Theophanides, T. (1993). Design and properties of maxillofacial prosthetic materials, *Med Device Technol*, *4*, 20-5.

[2] Cantor, R., Webber, R. L., Stroud, L. & Ryge, G. (1969). Methods for evaluating prosthetic facial materials. *J Prosthet Dent*, *21*, 324-332.

[3] Craig, R. G., Koran, A., Yu, R. & Spencer, J. (1978). Color stability of elastomers for maxillofacial appliances, *J Dent Res*, *57*, 866-871.

[4] Eleni, P. N., Katsavou, I., Krokida, M. K. & Polyzois, G. L. (2008). Color Stability of facial silicone prosthetic elastomers after artificial weathering. *Dent Res J*, *5*, 71-79.

[5] Gary, J. J. & Smith, C. T. (1998). Pigments and their application in maxillofacial elastomers: a literature review. *J Prosthet Dent*, *80*, 204-8.

[6] Guttal, S. S., Patil, N. P., Nadiger, R. K. & Kulkami, R. (2008). A study on reproduction silicone shade guide for maxillofacial prostheses matching Indian skin color. *Indian J Dent Res*, *19*, 191-5.

[7] Haddad, F. M., Goiato, C. M., Micheline Dos Santos, D., Moreno, A., Filipe D'almeida, N. & Alves Pesqueira, A. (2011). Color stability of maxillofacial silicone with nanoparticle pigment and opacifier submitted to disinfection and artificial aging. *J Biomed Opt*, *16*, 095004.

[8] Haddad, M. F., Goiato, M. C., Dos Santos, D. M., Pesqueira, A. A., Moreno, A. & Pellizzer, E. P. (2011). Influence of pigment and opacifier on dimensional stability and detail reproduction of maxillofacial silicone elastomer. *J Craniofac Surg*, *22*, 1612-1616.

[9] Haug, S. P., Andres, C. J. & Moore, B. K. (1999). Color stability and colorant effect on maxillofacial elastomers. Part III: weathering effect on color. *J Prosthet Dent*, *81*, 431-8.

[10] Judd, D. B. & Wyszecki, G. (1975). *Color in business, science and industry*. New York; Wiley & Sons Inc.

[11] Kiat-Amnuay, S., Johnston, D. A., Powers, J. M. & Jacob, R. F. (2005). Color stability of dry earth pigmented maxillofacial silicone a-2186 subjected to microwave energy exposur. *J Prosthodont*, *14*, 91-96.

[12] Lemon, J. C., Chambers, M. S., Jacobsen, M. L. & Powers, J. M. (1995). Color stability of facial prostheses. *J Prosthet Dent*, *74*, 613-618.

[13] Lewis, D. H. & Castleberry, D. J. (1980). An assessment of recent advances in external maxillofacial materials. *J Prosthet Dent*, *43*, 426-32.

[14] Sweeney, W. T., Fischer, T. E., Castleberry, D. J. & Cowperthwaite G. F. (1972). Evaluation of improved maxillofacial prosthetic materials. *J Prosthet Dent*, *27*, 297-305.

[15] Okubo, S. R., Kanawati, A., Richards, M. W. & Childress, S. (1998). Evaluation of visual and instrument shade matching. *I of Prosthet Dent*, *80*, 642-8.

[16] Over, L. M., Andres, C. J., Moore, B. K., Goodacre, C. J. & Muñoz, C. A. (1998). Using a colorimeter to develop an intrinsic silicone shade guide for facial prostheses. *J Prosthodont*, *7*, 237-49.

[17] Schaaf, N. G. (1970). Color characterizing silicone rubber facial prostheses. *J of Prosthet Dent*, *24*, 198-202.

[18] Sproull, R. C. (1973). Color matching in Dentistry Part I: The three dimensional nature of color. *J of Prosthet Dent*, *29*, 416-424.

[19] Sproull, R. C. (1973). Color matching in dentistry: Part II: Practical applications of the organization of color. *J of Prosthet Dent*, *29*, 556-566.

[20] Sproull, R. C. (1974). Color matching in dentistry. Part III: Color control. *J of Prosthet Dent*, *31*, 146-154.

[21] Turner, G. E., Fischer, T. E., Castleberry, D. J. & Lemons, J. E. (1984). Intrinsic color of isophorone polyurethane for maxillofacial prosthetics. Part II: Color Stability. *J Prosthet Dent*, *51*, 673-675.

[22] Zhou, H. F., Yu, W. & Yang, C. Y. (1998). A study of color matching of maxillofacial prosthesis. *Shangai Kou Qiang Yi Xue*, *7*, 25-7.

Chapter VI

The Aesthetics of Maxillofacial Prostheses

1. Aesthetics

The word "aesthetic" comes from the Greek words *aisthesis* or *aisthanesthai.* They mean "sense, to sense, senses, and to feel." The founder of modern aesthetics is Alexander G. Baumgarten. After the ancient period, many scientists have described aesthetics. Aristotle expressed that the symmetry and proportionality of materials forming a unity creates the proper aesthetic. According to Plato, good aesthetics consists of direct proportion. In order to qualify as aesthetics, it is necessary to not simply recognize a material by using visual senses, but also to evaluate it as beautiful, ugly, pretty, or not pretty [5, 8, 18, 36, 38].

The first region to give information about people and to be recognized first is the facial region. For these reasons, the face has always been significant historically. The mouth is one structure which significantly affects the appearance of the face. People regularly appeal to dentists to meet their aesthetic demands. For example, some people do not pay attention to the health and appearance of their rear teeth, but they do give attention to frontal decay, malformation, or shape problems and want them to be treated as soon as possible. The main motivation for this is to have a beautiful and attractive face because the facial region contributes, positively or negatively, to the self-esteem and self-respect of people, which cause people to feel better and also positive effects on social relationships and achieving life goals.

An aesthetically acceptable appearance constitutes the base of a healthy psychological structure. The human, the unity of his physical and psychological parts, always tries to balance them. One of the most important duties in this regard belongs to dentists. Here, the importance of the practice of aesthetic dentistry in human life appears.

Maxillofacial prostheses have a special place in dentistry terminology as the science and art of anatomical, functional, and cosmetic restoration of any region of maxilla, mandible, or any other region which has any defect due to surgical operation, trauma, pathology, congenital defect, or other reasons. Although materials and techniques have been widely developed in the past century, the first primitive maxillofacial prostheses were produced much earlier. Nasal, orbital, and auricular prostheses are seen on mummies from the 4th dynastic period of Egypt (1613-2494 B.C.), revealing that maxillofacial prostheses have been produced for thousands of years. It is also known that Chinese people have produced maxillofacial prostheses from paraffin and many other materials for many centuries. The French Surgeon Dentist Ambroise Pare is the first representative of the modern artificial eye. He produced an artificial ocular organ by using glass and porcelain in the year 1575. The contribution of dentistry to the development of an acrylic ocular organ is the production of ocular prostheses by measuring sockets rather than using traditional empirical methods. In the early 20th century, especially during and after the First World War, prostheses began to be produced with cooperation of surgeons and dentists.

Because the restoration of all the parts of the stomatognathic system and related environmental tissues with artificial materials and the reprovision of aesthetic results are very important for social adaptation and life quality, maxillofacial prostheses hold a very important place between all the classes of prosthetics.

Maxillofacial prostheses should restore lost tissues which cannot be rehabilitated by plastic surgery, including its color, shape, texture, and light transmittance, which must be in accord with near tissues. It should not be noticeable to society. A noticeable prosthesis increases the anxiety of the patient and it does not allow the desired social adaptation to occur. The aesthetic result at the end of the implementation of the prosthesis will bring clinical success [1, 12, 17, 21].

We should provide more basic information about this topic by expressing general aesthetic concepts of dentistry.

Aesthetic Concepts

1. **Composition:** When the contrast ratio of a material rises, its visibility also increases. Those can be contrasts on tissue, color, and line borders.
   The relationship between materials becoming visible through contrast is called composition.
2. **Unity:** The first condition of composition is to be unified. Unity makes the parts of the composition to be a single unit.
   There are two types of units:
   - **Static Units** are geometrical shapes with iterant figures, colors, and lines. For example, inorganic shapes, snow crystals, rain drops, and crystals are static units.
   - **Dynamic Units** are active, alive, and growing units existing in animals and plants.
3. **Cohesive and segregative forces:**
   Cohesive forces are the force which keep elements together in a certain form.
   Segregative Forces, in contrast with cohesive forces, allows many designs in unit.
   Both of these forces can be seen in dento-facial composition.
4. **Symmetry:** Symmetry refers to the order of the line of objects. There two types of symmetry:
   - **Horizontal symmetry** is the lining up of all of the elements with a certain distance from each other from left to right side.
   - **Radiational symmetry** is the lining up of objects as mirror images of each other at the two sides of central points.

   Both of these two types of symmetry are seen in dental line up.
5. **Proportion and Iterant Proportion:**
   Proportion is the mathematical expression of beauty and the numerical relationship between two parts.
   Iterant Proportion: When a surface is to be divided into parts with aesthetically different volumes and shapes, there must be a numeric proportion between them.
6. **Balance** is the arrangement of all the parts in such a way that none of them would be conspicuous and they would be equal to each other. As a result, there is a stabilization occurring by balancing contrary forces. Our visual sense is accustomed to providing this balance.

7. **Lines:** The most compatible structure consists of two parallel lines. The most powerful visual relationship is orthogonal lines. That is why the symbol of (=) is used for equilibrium and the symbol of (+) is used for a powerful relationship.
8. **Dominance** is a necessity for a unit. Color, shape, and lines may be a factor of dominance. It expresses the existence of a similar element continuing in the unit. That gives a dynamic structure to the composition.

2. The Principles of Structural Aesthetics

1. Facial Components

The human face can be divided into three parts in terms of a frontal perspective:

- trichion (hairy skin) and supraorbital region
- supraorbital and nasion (nasal base)
- nasal base and gnathion (the edge of chin) region

When the lips are closed, the face can be divided by a line from upper side of upper lip, whereby the bottom part of face constitutes 1/3 of the total face.

When looking at the face from the top, it can be concave, convex, or flat in accordance with lines passing on glabellas where the start point is the upper lip and chin edge.

a. Facial specifications

Indicators of aging start to be seen around the 25th year of life. These indicators gains speed between the 35th and 40th years of life. In general, there is water loss in cells and increasing fibrosis in all tissues and organs. As a result, the epidermis slims and skin rugae start due to the lack of elastin and collagen in the skin.

After the 60th year of life, the nasal edge, chin edge, and brows begin to lean out due to the effects of gravity. The nasal base falls down. The chin edge looks like it would touch with the nasal. The mouth edges lean out. Because of a decrease in vertical height, the vermillion line's width decreases and lips become indistinct.

Considering facial aging, the most affected region of the face is the lower 1/3 portion. This region is surrounded by anatomic facial sulcuses. Those are nasolabial, labial, and mentolabial sulcuses. The loss of dento-alveolar support in muscles under those sulcuses leads them to lose their physiological lengths and their tonicity decreases. Finally, those sulcuses become deeper.

Middle Line

Although the right and left halves of the face looks symmetrical, there are some differences between its two halves. If the mirror image of one part is placed on other side, the resulting image will not be a natural appearance. For example, eyes have slightly different levels and depths in the eye socket. Also, for many people, nasal and chin edges may deviate according to a middle line.

But those shape, volume, and color differences cannot be recognized by the naked eye.

b. The Golden Rule

Pythagoras found a formula in order to express beauty in terms of different lengths and proportions as follows:

$$\frac{\text{Short Edge}}{\text{Long Edge}} = \frac{\text{Long Edge}}{\text{Long+ Short Edge}} = \frac{2}{15} = 0.618$$

The Golden Ratio has been widely used in art and architecture. That ratio exists in nature as well as the human body. It is also known as the "Holy Ratio." Our eyes are familiar with the golden ratio and our aesthetic preferences are in accordance with that familiarity.

Middle Line

Studies show that the best visual reference on the face is the philtrum. While the maxillary middle line and facial middle line keep going together by 70%, maxillary and mandibular lines keep separating by 75%. Accordingly, the dental middle line is the line which virtually divides maxillary central teeth. So, it passes through nasion and philtrum bases.

Although the face looks symmetrical, there are some differences between its two halves. If the mirror image of one part is placed on the other side, the resulting image will not be a natural appearance. For example, eyes have slightly different levels and depths in the eye socket. Also, for many people, nasal and chin edges may deviate according to the middle line [5, 8, 18, 20, 22, 25-27, 33, 35, 38-40].

3. Aesthetics of Maxillofacial Prostheses

a. Aesthetics of Auricular Prostheses

While auricular defects may be reconstructed by using autogenous tissues, an appropriate prosthetic reconstruction using a suitable material is a quick and affordable solution for a natural or almost natural appearance.

Additionally, it requires no surgical operation in order to achieve cohesiveness and retention, except a first surgery for preparation of the defect region.

Although there are many techniques for preparation and positioning of the prosthesis morphology to be similar with the other ear and for its adaptation to tissues in the defect region, those methods depend on the talent of the technician and they carry a high risk of failure. To prepare an ear prosthesis prototype and to achieve the mirror image of the ear, the use of CT, KIBT, optic systems, and laser surface scanners, CAD, CNC and fast prototyping techniques is very advantageous. CT data are also very useful for correct positioning of prosthesis.

The paraffin prosthesis sample must be controlled on the patient in terms of some rules of aesthetics and compliance, position, slope, and level. The references used in this phase are anatomic landmarks such as the hair line, mandible angle, and mastoid bump.

Also, the guidance of vertical and horizontal orientation lines are used. The top height of the helix should be controlled by comparing it with the normal ear. The upper lines of helixes and lower lines of both the ears should be on the same horizontal line. Another helpful reference point is the distance between the back of ear and cranium. Considering those rules, the paraffin sample is controlled on the patient. After appropriate compliances, the prosthesis is finished by giving tissue characterizations to the paraffin sample [1, 9, 23, 26, 29, 42].

Because the location of the implant to be placed on the temporal region in an implant reinforced auricular prosthesis is also aesthetically important, the placement of retention systems in the borders of auricular prosthesis should be at the same level as the anti-helix. Implants must be 7mm away from hairy skin and 15mm away from each other. By taking the width of the outer ear on mastoid bone as a reference, implants must be placed on a line 18-22mm away from the canal. Locations between 9-11 o'clock for the right ear and 2-3 o'clock for the left ear are appropriate for implant placement.

Creating a completely adopted frontal line for auricular prosthesis is aesthetically important. It may lead to confusion in cases of mimics, head posture, mandible movements, facial asymmetry, and finally aesthetic. While those problems can be generally solved by randomly digging the frontal border of a master model, desired results may not be always achieved because this implementation is not a controlled method. The distance occurring on the frontal border due to the movements of the chin and head can be solved by providing a barrier on the frontal region of the master model and by elastically preparing the frontal border of the prosthesis. The digging of the model should be preceded by a clinical evaluation of the soft tissues.

b. Aesthetics of Nasal Prostheses

The implementation of nasal prostheses can be started 4-6 months after surgery. The size and shape of the defect are very important for the success of prostheses. A prosthesis is more successful in cases protected by nasolabial sulcus. Because most of the lower border tissues in nasal defects are mobile, prostheses must be prepared as elastic and as thin as possible in those regions.

The main factors affecting the aesthetic success of prostheses are appropriate creation of contours, masking demarcation lines, and compliance of the prosthesis surface and the skin. The width of nasal wings must be prepared in such a way as to not exceed the distance between the inner edges of the eyes. Also, the conjunction of columella and skin must be finished as narrow and perpendicular so the demarcation line will be less visible because of the shade of the nasal edge. For male patients, this region can also be masked by adding a mustache. Eyeglasses are used for masking the demarcation lines in lateral and upper regions and for retention purposes.

Considering the color loss during painting and finishing phases, the painting must be performed slightly more significantly than the near skin. After final controls and corrections on the patient, the finishing stage begins [2, 4, 6, 10, 13, 15, 16, 21, 28, 30-34].

c. Aesthetics of Orbital Prostheses

Prostheses made for the restoration of upper and lower eyelids, inner and outer canthi, and tissues extending from the orbita through the face, except eyeball, are considered orbital or oculo-facial prostheses. Because communication between people generally begins with eye contact and the position of the eyes, the contour of the eyelids and even minimal differences in the colors of the prosthesis can be discerned easily, making aesthetic success very important.

It is important to take care of orbital prostheses by masking borders and artificiality by preparing it in accordance with the structure and color of healthy tissues. Besides skin properties, the symmetry of synthetic eyebrows and lashes in terms of color, thickness, and shape is also important for aesthetic success. Also, the preparation of the prosthesis with borders as thin as possible, in a way which does not break the harmony of the mimicry, should be considered. The most frequently used camouflage method for borders of these prostheses is the usage of thick eyeglass with light colored lenses. The rugae and lines around eye are exploited in old patients. In cases where surgical resection exceeds the border of the orbita, some aesthetic problems increase due to the failure to mask the conjunction regions between skin and prosthesis.

In order to produce an adequately compliant prosthesis, the measurement must be performed for the entire face. With developments in digital technology, the measurements of the facial region are performed by fast prototyping the data acquired from laser surface scanners and optical systems by using CAD&CAM, without measuring the face manually. Then, a model is created. Because this method records tissues in a static state, the adaptation in conjunction points can be broken with movement, and movements can be limited with pain [13, 14, 23, 24, 42].

The placement of the ocular part of orbital prosthesis at the same level as the healthy eye in terms of horizontal, vertical, and sagittal axes is very important for aesthetic success. While the patient looks directly at a far point when he stands tall, the ocular part of prosthesis must be placed inside of the defect in such a way as to imitate that look. After the ocular part is located with the assistance of horizontal and vertical drawings and measurements, then the eyelid contour of the healthy eye is drawn on the prosthesis by using paraffin.

Computerized monitoring techniques may be used for determining the correct ocular and eyelid position. For this purpose, a digital image of the patient is created by a digital camera from lens-object distance and the mirror image of healthy region is reflected over the orbital defect region with a software package such as Adobe Photoshop. After a cut-paste process by taking images of the paraffin model, where the ocular part placed, from object-lens distance, the image of the healthy eye is placed on the prosthesis. Through that image, the position of the ocular part and eyelids can be controlled. After providing correct positioning, the paraffin sample is given skin properties by correcting contours and borders. Then it is finished by coloring and shading through the use of silicon material. While retention can be provided by using adhesives, tissue undercuts, eyeglasses, and implants for most cases, implants are preferred more for large defects such that the resection is on the cheek or other mobile tissues.

d. Aesthetics of Mid-facial Defects

The treatment of advanced tumors in the middle region of the face generally requires very large tissue resection. The defects in such kinds of cases include the loss of intra-oral and extra-oral tissues together. Nasal, upper lip, cheek, or orbital structures may be included in that lost of tissue. Also, mandible, soft tissues, teeth, and segments of the maxilla may be lost. Functional losses can be very advanced as a result of such kinds of surgical resections. The loss of the oral cavity may lead to malfunctions in chewing, swallowing, saliva control, and speaking. With cosmetic losses, those functional losses create serious psychological trauma in patients and their relatives. However, because of the development of materials and techniques in recent years, patients with such kinds of defects can be successfully rehabilitated through prosthetic restorations.

The monoblock prosthesis is preferred for the restoration of large maxillofacial defects, including cheek regions and orbital-nasal regions, not including the lip and oral cavity.

The usage of cranio-facial and zygomatic implants is very important for retention of those prostheses. In order to provide the retention of large prosthetic restorations, the use of adhesives and tissue undercuts is almost impossible.

Secondary surgical procedures may be required for those defects or there may be significant contour failures, asymmetries, or skin discoloration due to radiotherapy. For the best results, the contours and surface structures of the prosthesis must be in accordance with those of the patient's skin. The compliance of the prosthetic surface with the patient's skin is very important. Intra-oral and extra-oral prostheses are generally used in combination for mid-facial defects. Generally, the aesthetic desires are not as important for those patients as the need for filling the defect. In such cases, sensitive retentioners are used for only retention indication without any aesthetic purpose in treatments of intra-oral defects.

However, after uncomplicated maxillectomy implementations, sensitive retentioners are used for providing both aesthetics and retention by eliminating buccal clasp booms [17, 21, 29].

REFERENCES

[1] Andreopoulos, A. G. & Theophanides, T. (1993). Design and properties of maxillofacial prosthetic materials, *Med Device Technol*, *4*, 20-5.

[2] Aydınatay, K., Korkmaz, T., Coşkun, A., Yılmaz, C. & Yaluğ, S. (2004). Analysis of heat caused change colored and noncolored maxillofacial elastomers. *J of Dental Faculty of Cumhuriyet University*, *7*, 11-19.

[3] Cantor, R., Webber, R. L., Stroud, L. & Ryge, G. (1969). Methods for evaluating prosthetic facial materials. *J of Prosthet Dent*, *21*, 324-332.

[4] Craig, R. G., Koran, A., Yu, R. & Spencer, J. (1978). Color stability of elastomers for maxillofacial appliances *J Dent Res*, *57*, 866-871.

[5] Espesito, S. C. (1980). Esthetics for denture patients. *J Prosthetic Dentistry*, *44*, 608-615.

[6] Eleni, P. N., Katsavou, I., Krokida, M. K. & Polyzois, G. L. (2008). Color Stability of facial silicone prosthetic elastomers after artificial weathering. *Dent Res J*, *5*, 71-79.

[7] Gary, J. J. & Smith, C. T. (1998). Pigments and their application in maxillofacial elastomers: A literature review. *J Prosthet Dent*, *80*, 204-8.

[8] Goldstein, R. E. (1976). *Esthetics in Dentistry*. Atlanta; Lippincott Co.

[9] Guttal, S. S., Patil, N. P., Nadiger, R. K. & Kulkami, R. (2008). A study on reproduction silicone shade guide for maxillofacial prostheses matching Indian skin color. *Indian J Dent Res*, *19*, 191-5.

[10] Haddad, F. M., Goiato, C. M., Micheline Dos Santos, D., Moreno, A., Filipe D'almeida, N. & Alves Pesqueira, A. (2011). Color stability of maxillofacial silicone with nanoparticle pigment and opacifier submitted to disinfection and artificial aging. *J Biomed Opt*, *16*, 095004.

[11] Haddad, M. F., Goiato, M. C., Dos Santos, D. M., Pesqueira, A. A., Moreno, A. & Pellizzer, E. P. (2011). Influence of pigment and opacifier on dimensional stability and detail reproduction of maxillofacial silicone elastomer. *J Craniofac Surg*, *22*, 1612-1616.

[12] Hanson, M. D., Shipman, B., Blomfield, J. V. & Janus, C. E. (1983). Commercial cosmetics and their role in the coloring of facial prostheses. *J of Prosthet Dent*, *50*, 818-820.

[13] Haug, S. P., Andres, C. J. & Moore, B. K. (1999). Color stability and colorant effect on maxillofacial elastomers. Part III: weathering effect on color. *J of Prosthet Dent*, *81*, 431-8.

[14] Judd, D. B. & Wyszecki, G. (1975). *Color in business, science and industry*. New York; Wiley & Sons Inc.

[15] Kiat-Amnuay, S., Johnston, D. A., Powers, J. M. & Jacob, R. F. (2005). Color stability of dry earth pigmented maxillofacial silicone a-2186 subjected to microwave energy exposur. *J Prosthodont*, *14*, 91-96.

[16] Lemon, J. C., Chambers, M. S., Jacobsen, M. L. & Powers, J. M. (1995). Color stability of facial prostheses. *J of Prosthet Dent*, *74*, 613-618.

[17] Lewis, D. H. & Castleberry, D. J. (1980). An assessment of recent advances in external maxillofacial materials. *J of Prosthet Dent*, *43*, 426-32.

[18] Maruyama, T. (1998). Esthetic dentistry in the twenty-first century. *Dental Clinics of North America*, *42*, 695-711.

[19] Miller, A., Long, J., Cole, J. & Staffanou, R. (1993). Shade selection and laboratory communication. *Quintessence Inter*, *24*, 305-309.

[20] Morley, J. (2001). Macroesthetic Elements of Smile Design. *JADA*, *132*, 39-45.

[21] Murat, S., Gürbüz, A., Günay, Y. & Oruç, A. S. (2011). Aesthetic approaches in maxillofacial prosthesis. *J Dental Sci-Special Topics*, *2*, 97-114.

[22] Neumann, L. M., Christensen, C. & Cavanaugh, C. (1989). Dental esthetic satisfaction in adults. *JADA*, *118*, 565-569.

[23] Okubo, S. R., Kanawati, A., Richards, M. W. & Childress, S. (1998). Evaluation of visual and instrument shade matching. *J of Prosthet Dent*, *80*, 642-8.

[24] Over, L. M., Andres, C. J., Moore, B. K., Goodacre, C. J. & Muñoz, C. A. (1998). Using a colorimeter to develop an intrinsic silicone shade guide for facial prostheses. *J Prosthodont*, *7*, 237-49.

[25] Pogrel, M. A. (1991). What are normal esthetic value? *J Oral Maxillofac Surgery*, *49*, 963-969.

[26] Rahn, A. O. & Boucher, L. J. (1970). *Maxillofacial prosthetics principles and consepts*. Philedalphia; W.B. Saunders Company.

[27] Rufenacht, C. R. (1990). *Fundamental of Esthetics*. Hardcover; Quintessence Pub.

[28] Schaaf, N. G. (1970). Color characterizing silicone rubber facial prostheses. *J of Prosthet Dent*, *24*,198-202.

[29] Sweeney, W. T., Fischer, T. E., Castleberry, D. J. & Cowperthwaite G. F. (1972). Evaluation of improved maxillofacial prosthetic materials. *J of Prosthet Dent*, *27*, 297-305.

[30] Sproull, R. C. (1973). Color matching in Dentistry Part I: The three dimensional nature of color. *J of Prosthet Dent*, *29*, 416-424.

[31] Sproull, R. C. (1973). Color matching in dentistry: Part II: Practical applications of the organization of color. *J of Prosthet Dent*, *29*, 556-566.

[32] Sproull, R. C. (1974). Color matching in dentistry. Part III: Color control. *J of Prosthet Dent*, *31*, 146-154.

[33] Touyz, L. Z. G. & Harel-Raviv, M. (1999). Cosmetic or esthetic dentistry? *Quintessence Inter*, *30*, 227-233.

[34] Turner, G. E., Fischer, T. E., Castleberry, D. J. & Lemons, J. E. (1984). Intrinsic color of isophorone polyurethane for maxillofacial prosthetics. Part II: Color Stability. *J of Prosthet Dent*, *51*, 673-675.

[35] Sorensen, J. A., Newman, M. G. & Flemming, T. F. (1991). Gingival enhancement in fixed prosthodontics. Part I: Clinical findings. *J Prosthetic Dent*, *65*, 100-107.

[36] Strub, J. R. & Turp, J. C. (1999). *Esthetics and Dental Prosthetic.* Chicago; Quintessence.

[37] Suman, T. (2011). Enhancing facial esthetics by other modalities. *Int J Dent.* 513957. doi: 10.1155/2011/513957.

[38] Tjan, A. H. & Miller, G. D. (1984). Some aesthetic factors in a smile. *J Prosthetic Dent*, *51*, 24-28.

[39] Tripodakis, A. P. (1987). Dental esthetics: Oral personality and visual perception. *Quintessence Inter*, *18*, 405-418.

[40] Ward, D. H. (2001). Proportional smile design using the recurring esthetic dental (RED) proportion. *Dental Clinics of North America*, *45*, 143-153.

[41] Zhou, H. F., Yu, W. & Yang, C. Y. (1998). A study of color matching of maxillofacial prosthesis. *Shangai Kou Qiang Yi Xue*, *7*, 25-7.

[42] Zyl, I. V. & Geissberger, M. (2001). Simulated shape design. *JADA*, *132*, 1105-1109.

Chapter VII

THE PROCESS OF COPING WITH PROSTHESES FOR DEFECT PATIENTS

The choice of the rehabilitation of maxillofacial defects by surgical or prosthetic methods depends on the patient's desires as well as the size and etiology of defects. While young patients usually desire their facial region to be treated with their own tissues rather than prostheses, older patients usually desire to be treated by using prostheses [2, 7, 11, 30, 36]. Generally, small maxillofacial defects are treated by surgical methods, while larger defects are treated by prosthetic restorations in order to give a more natural appearance. This process requires more complicated procedures. Patients with those kinds of defects are generally older patients and may not be able to tolerate those kinds of treatments.

Also, the radiation used for the treatment of tumors, which are the causes of these defects, may lead vascularity to decrease, fibrosis to increase, complications to occur, and the surgery area to not heal after surgical operation. Additionally, if any defect area appeared after the removal of a tumor, the prosthetic treatment of the defect area allows the region to be closely and frequently monitored in terms of the risk of recurrence. Factors such as the age of the patient, the defect area's largeness which does not allow the area to be able to close by surgical methods, the patient's risk of recurrence, and the need to be frequently monitored determine the prosthesis planning [2, 8].

Acrylic resins, polyurethane elastomers, and silicone elastomers are used for the production of current maxillofacial prosthesis. Some of the advantages of acrylic resins are their acceptable physical and chemical resistances, familiarity of most of doctors with their production, their ability to be painted from both inside and outside, their ability to provide a thin passage on borders between the defect area and the prosthesis, and their harmony with most adhesive systems. They have also some disadvantages, including the fact that they have no elasticity (elasticity is demanded for most patients), their lack of compliance with mobile tissues, discomfort caused by irritation of tissues, and high thermal conductance. Besides the advantages of polyurethane elastomers, such as their ability to be thinned at their edges without any laceration or enlargement or any harm, they have also some disadvantages, such as high moisture sensitivity of the isocyanate included in them, not having color stability, not being compatible with adhesive systems, and the toxicity of isocyanate. Silicone elastomers are the most used materials for maxillofacial prostheses. Most of those materials have little resistance against laceration and their painting procedures are very difficult. The resistance against laceration is higher in RTVs (silicone vulcanizing at room temperature) and HTVs (silicone vulcanizing by heating). But because of their easy usage, natural results when they are colored, successful shaping, color stability, ease to clean, and (most importantly) not having harmful elasticity, and being compatible with mobile tissue regions, RTVs are generally preferred for the restoration of defect regions [8, 11, 26].

One of the most significant problems associated with maxillofacial prostheses is the lack of stability and retention. Retention is provided through adhesive systems, mechanic methods, tissues in anatomical areas, and also implants. Adhesive bands, aromatic cements, and silicone-based adhesives are used as adhesive systems. Because of daily relocation of adhesive bands, undesired edge loss of a prosthesis may occur and there may be problems in the adhesion of the band to silicon. Daily extraction of adhesive cements may be harmful for the surface color of prostheses and may lead to edge loss. Silicone solvent is required for cleaning silicone adhesives. Those solvents may lead to the preservation of elasticity and extend the value of the material to change. Because of such kinds of limitations, restorations cannot provide perfect function and aesthetics, and they need to be changed periodically. On the other hand, tissue barriers also cannot provide perfect retention. So, osseo-integrated implants offer much better retention [2, 4, 5, 7-10, 13, 18, 26, 27].

QUALITY OF LIFE OF DEFECT PATIENTS

In recent years, there has been growing interest in using patient-reported outcomes in order to facilitate patient-centered care, to screen for physical and psychological problems, and to monitor a patient's progress over time. Facial disfigurement as a result of a congenital anomaly, trauma, or tumor surgery can have devastating effects on the aesthetic, functional, economic, and psychosocial aspects of a person's life [1, 3, 5, 12, 14, 15, 22, 31, 32, 34, 39, 40, 44-46].

Patients with maxillofacial defects may express unhappiness with their body image, often leading to low self-esteem, post-traumatic stress disorder symptoms, and social isolation caused by stigma. Stigma is accepted as an important social determinant of health because it may contribute to suffering, delay in appropriate help-seeking, treatment dropout, and treatment effectiveness. Thus, stigma has become a matter of particular interest for public health. In this context, maxillofacial rehabilitation through prosthetic restoration is a cornerstone of efforts to restore the function and form of patients with missing or disfigured facial structures. Maxillofacial prosthetics, as an alternative to surgery, offer non-operative rehabilitation, seeking to provide satisfactory aesthetics and quality of life (QOL), and thus to facilitate reinstatement of patients in their family situations and social environments. Previous studies have shown that patients with acquired facial disfigurement have greater psychosocial problems, difficulty adjusting to their facial disfigurement, and more physical impairment of QOL than patients with congenital facial disfigurement. Because of this, in a clinical setting, the identification of the need for prosthetic rehabilitation in these patients, a process which can restore QOL, is most important. Recent studies have emphasized the importance of developing additional programs to improve the quality of care and to enhance the well-being and satisfaction of patients. The evaluation of patients' QOL related to prosthetic rehabilitation may provide valuable information to assist the maxillofacial prosthodontic team in treatment planning, monitoring, and outcome assessment. Although there is much research regarding the effects of prosthetic rehabilitation on health-related QOL in patients with maxillary defects, there are few studies investigating the health-related QOL of adult patients with facial prostheses. Recent data shows that implant-retained maxillofacial prostheses provided a significant enhancement in patients' QOL and that they were tolerated more easily than adhesively-retained prostheses [5, 8, 10, 18, 38]. Patients with acquired orbital and nasal defects had lower health-related QOL than healthy individuals, as well as patients with acquired auricular defects.

Health-related QOL is a multi-dimensional global construct, defined as an individual's perception of his or her position in life, in the context of the culture and value systems in which the person lives and in relation to that individual's goals, expectations, standards, and concerns. Patients' perceptions of treatment with maxillofacial prostheses are key elements in evaluating quality of care, because measuring patient outcomes, such as health-related QOL, in clinical practice may provide important information for planning and evaluation of extensive maxillofacial prosthetic rehabilitation [2, 12, 14, 17, 21, 22, 24, 25, 27, 33, 39, 40, 41, 44, 45].

It is known that the loss of part of the face and its prosthetic restoration requires social and psychological adjustment because a visible disfigurement leads to lowered self-esteem, negative self-image and social isolation for life [16, 6, 25, 28, 29, 35, 42, 43, 46]. Klein et al. [22] showed that the patient's own body image is significantly altered without a restriction in the acceptance of their body by others. Newton et al. [30] reported that these patients experienced many psychological and social problems, such as negative feelings or avoiding showing their partner their face, without the prosthesis. The adjustment process to disfiguring conditions and maxillofacial prostheses are influenced by the interaction between various underlying cognitive self-schemas, and the social and cultural context. This may be explained by the fact that people with impaired vision had serious restrictions in physical activities (reading, outdoor mobility, participation in leisure activities, and shopping) that were negatively related to the experience of health and vitality[5, 6, 16, 19, 20, 23, 43]. In addition, monocular vision and the associated compromise in depth perception may reduce the patient's ability to clean their prosthesis with hygiene products and the quality of their hygiene. Patients with prosthetic noses reported more problems with the prostheses, such as going out in hot and cold weather, playing sports, and allergies, that affect their psychological and social well-being. Other possible explanations for this can be drawn from our experiences that these patients experience difficulties in camouflaging the scars and prosthesis margins more than other patients.

References

[1] Ahn, J. M., Lee, S. Y. & Yoon, J. S. (2010). Health-related quality of life and emotional status of anophthalmic patients in Korea. *Am J Ophthalmol, 149*, 1005-11.

[2] Anderson, J. D. & Szalai, J. P. (2003). The Toronto outcome measure for craniofacial prosthetics: a condition-specific quality-of-life instrument. *Int J Oral Maxillofac Implants*, *18*, 531-8.

[3] Biordi, D. & Nicholson, N. (2008). *Social Isolation. In Chronic Illness Impact and Interventions.*7th edition. Edited by Larsen, P. Boston, MA; Jones & Bartlett Publishing, Inc; 85-115.

[4] Bonanno, A. & Choi, J. Y. (2011). Psychosocial aspects of orbitofacial disfigurement in cancer patients. *Ophthalmic Oncology* (M.D. Anderson Solid Tumor Oncology Series), *6*, 311-8.

[5] Bou, C., Pomar, P., Miquel, J. L. & Poisson, P. (2006). Maxillo-facial prostheses: an issue in public health. *Odontostomatol Trop*, *29*, 34-40.

[6] Cağlayan, D. (2008). *The Attitudes of Responsible Local Agencies Towards Disability*. PhD thesis. Middle East Technical University, Ankara, The Graduate School of Natural And Applied Sciences.

[7] Callahan, C. (2004). Facial disfigurement and sense of self in head and neck cancer. *Soc Work Health Care*, *40*, 73-87.

[8] Chang, T. L., Garrett, N., Roumanas, E. & Beumer, III. J. (2005). Treatment satisfaction with facial prostheses. *J Prosthet Dent*, *94*, 275-80.

[9] Cheng, A. C., Leong, E. W., Khin, N. T., Wee, A. G., Fung, C. K. & Lee, C. M. (2007). Osseointegrated implants in craniofacial application: current status. *Singapore Dent J*, *29*, 1-11.

[10] De Sousa, A. (2008). Psychological issues in oral and maxillofacial reconstructive surgery. *British J of Oral and Maxillofac Surg*, *46*, 661-4.

[11] De Sousa, A. (2010). Psychological issues in acquired facial trauma. *Indian J Plast Surg*, *43*, 200-5.

[12] Depprich, R., Naujoks, C., Lind, D., Ommerborn, M., Meyer, U., Kübler, N. R. & Handschel, J. (2011). Evaluation of the quality of life of patients with maxillofacial defects after prosthodontic therapy with obturator prostheses. *Int J Oral Maxillofac Surg*, *40*, 71-9.

[13] Dostalova, T., Kozak, J., Hubacek, M., Holakovsky, J., Kr, P., Starnad, J. & Seydlova, M. (2011). Facial prosthesis: In implant dentistry - A rapidly evolving practice. In Turkyilmaz I. Editor. (451- 64). Croatia, InTech.

[14] Dos Santos, D. M., Goiato, M. C., Pesqueira, A. A., Bannwart, L. C., Rezende, M. C., Magro-Filho, O. & Moreno, A. (2010). Prosthesis auricular with osseointegrated implants and quality of life. *J Craniofac Surg.*, *21*, 94-6.

[15] Eser, E., Fidaner, H., Fidaner, C., Eser, S. Y., Elbi, H. & Göker, E. (1999). Psychometric properties of WHOQOL-100 and WHOQOLBREF. *J Psychiatr Psychol Psychopharmacol*, *7*, 23–40.

[16] Fırat, S. (2010). People with disabilities in Turkey: An overview. *Information technologies, Management and Society*, *3*, 51-4.

[17] Genden, E. M., Okay, D., Stepp, M. T., Rezaee, R. P., Mojica, J. S., Buchbinder, D. & Urken, M. L. (2003). Comparison of functional and quality-of-life outcomes in patients with and without palatomaxillary reconstruction: a preliminary report. *Arch Otolaryngol Head Neck Surg*, *129*, 775-80.

[18] Goiato, M. C., Pesqueira, A. A., Ramos da Silva, C., Gennari Filho, H. & Micheline Dos Santos, D. (2009). Patient satisfaction with maxillofacial prosthesis. Literature review. *J Plast Reconstr Aesthet Surg*, *62*, 175-80.

[19] Horlock, N., Vogelin, E., Bradbury, E. T., Grobbelaar, A. O. & Gault, D. T. (2005). Psychosocial outcome of patients after ear reconstruction: a retrospective study of 62 patients. *Ann Plast Surg*, *54*, 517-24.

[20] Immerman, S., Constantinides, M., Pribitkin, E. A. & White W. M. (2010). Nasal soft tissue trauma and management. *Facial Plast Surg*, *26*, 522-31.

[21] Irish, J., Sandhu, N., Simpson, C., Wood, R., Gilbert, R., Gullane, P., Brown, D., Goldstein, D., Devins, G. & Barker, E. (2009). Quality of life in patients with maxillectomy prostheses. *Head Neck*, *31*, 813-21.

[22] Klein, M., Menneking, H., Spring, A. & Rose, M. (2005). Analysis of quality of life in patients with a facial prosthesis. *Mund Kiefer Gesichtschir*, *9*, 205-13.

[23] Kock, M. (2004). Disability Law in Germany: An Overview of Employment, Education and Access Rights GLJ, *5*, 1373-92.

[24] Kornblith, A. B., Zlotolow, I. M., Gooen, J., Huryn, J. M., Lerner, T., Strong, E. W., Shah, J. P., Spiro, R. H. & Holland, J. C. (1996). Quality of life of maxillectomy patients using an obturators prosthesis. *Head Neck*, *18*, 323-34.

[25] Levine, E., Degutis, L., Pruzinsky, T., Shin, J. & Persing, J. A. (2005). Quality of life and facial trauma: psychological and body image effects. *Ann Plast Surg*, *54*, 502-10.

[26] Leonardi, A., Buonaccorsi, S., Pellacchia, V., Moricca, L. M., Indrizzi, E. & Fini, G. (2008). Maxillofacial prosthetic rehabilitation using extraoral implants. *J Craniofac Surg*, *19*, 398- 405.

[27] Lohr, K. N. & Zebrack, B. J. (2009). Using patient-reported outcomes in clinical practice: challenges and opportunities. *Qual Life Res*, *18*, 99-107.

[28] Lim, S. Y., Lee, D., Oh, K. S., Nam, B., Bang, S. I., Mun, G. H., Pyon, J. K., Kim, J. H., Yoon, C. S., Song, H. S. & Jeon, H. J. (2010). Concealment, depression and poor quality of life in patients with congenital facial anomalies. *J Plast Reconstr Aesth Surg*, *63*, 1982-89.

[29] Murphy, B. A., Ridner, S., Wells, N. & Dietrich, M. (2007). Quality of life research in head and neck cancer: a review of the current state of the science. *Crit Rev Oncol Hematol*, *62*, 251-67.

[30] Newton, J. T., Fiske, J., Foote, O., Frances, C., Loh, I. M. & Radford, D. R. (1999). Preliminary study of the impact of loss of part of the face and its prosthetic restoration. *J Prosthet Dent*, *82*, 585-90.

[31] Patrick, D. L. & Deyo, R. A. (1989). Generic and disease-specific measures in assessing health status and quality of life. *Med Care*, *27*, 217-32.

[32] Pine, K., Sloan, B., Stewart, J. & Jacobs, R. J. (2011). Concerns of anophthalmic patients wearing artificial eyes. *Clin Experiment Ophthalmol*, *39*, 47-52.

[33] Riaz, N. & Warriach, R. A. (2010). Quality of life in patients with obturator prostheses. *J Ayub Med Coll Abbottabad*, *22*, 121-5.

[34] Robinson, E. (1997). *Psychological research on visible differences in adults.* In Visibly different: Coping with disfigurement. In: Lansdown R., Editor, Rumsey N. Editor, Bradbury E. Editor, Carr T. Editor, Partridge J. Editor, Butterworth-Heinemann Oxford; 102–11.

[35] Rumsey, N. & Harcourt, D. (2004). Body image and disfigurement: issues and interventions. *Body Image*, *1*, 83-97.

[36] Saka, Ö. & Varol, N. (2007). Institutional and community care for older people in Turkey. *Eurohealth*, *13*, 20-2.

[37] Skevington, S. M., Lotfy, M., O'Connell, K. A. & WHOQOL Group (2004). The world health organization's WHOQOL-BREF quality of life assessment: psychometric properties and results of the international field trial. A report from the WHOQOL group. *Qual Life Res*, *13*, 299–310.

[38] Schoen, P. J., Raghoebar, G. M., van Oort, R. P., Reintsema. H., van der Laan, B. F., Burlage, F. R., Roodenburg, J. L. & Vissink, A. (2001). Treatment outcome of bone-anchored craniofacial prostheses after tumor surgery. *Cancer*, *92*, 3045-50.

[39] Sloan, J. A., Tolman, D. E., Anderson, J. D., Sugar, A. W., Wolfaardt, J. F. & Novotny, P. (2001). Patients with reconstruction of craniofacial or intra-oral defects: Development of instruments to measure quality of life. *Int J Oral Maxillofac Implants*, *16*, 225–45.

[40] Snyder, C. F., Aaronson, N. K., Choucair, A. K., 6 Elliott, T. E., Greenhalgh, J., Halyard, M. Y., Hess, R., Miller, D. M., Reeve, B. B. & Santana, M. (2012). Implementing patient-reported outcomes assessment in clinical practice: a review of the options and considerations. *Qual Life Res*, *21*, 1305-14.

[41] Streiner, D. L. & Norman, G. R. (1991). *Health measurement scales: a practical guide to their development and use*. New York. Oxford University Press.

[42] Thompson, A. & Kent, G. (2001). Adjusting to disfigurement: processes involved in dealing with being visibly different. *Clin Psychol Rev*, *21*, 663-82.

[43] Weiss, M. G., Ramakrishna, J. & Somma, D. (2006). Health-related stigma: Rethinking concepts and interventions. *Psychol Health Med*, *11*, 277 – 87.

[44] WHOQOL Group (1994). Development of the WHOQOL: Rationale and current status. *Int J Mental Health*, *23*, 24-56.

[45] WHOQOL Group (1998). Development of the WHOQOL: WHOQOL-BREF quality of life assessment. *Psychol Med*, *28*, 551–8.

[46] Versnel, S. L., Plomp, R. G., Passchier, J., Duivenvoorden, H. J. & Mathijssen, I. M. (2012). Long-term psychological functioning of adults with severe congenital facial disfigurement. *Plast Reconstr Surg*, *129*, 110-117.

EDITOR CONTACT INFORMATION

Dr. Arzu Atay
Associate Professor
Department of Prosthodontics
GATA Haydarpasa Training Hospital
Istanbul, Turkey
Tel: +0905053992373
Fax: +902165422020
arzuatay@gmail.com

INDEX

G

H

I

J

K

L

M

N

O

P

T

U

V

W

Y

Z